Genetics of Cardiac Arrhythmias

Guest Editor

SILVIA G. PRIORI, MD, PhD

CARDIAC ELECTROPHYSIOLOGY CLINICS

www.cardiacEP.theclinics.com

Consulting Editors

RANJAN K. THAKUR, MD, MPH, MBA, FHRS
ANDREA NATALE, MD, FACC, FHRS

December 2010 • Volume 2 • Number 4

SAUNDERS an imprint of ELSEVIER, Inc.

W.B. SAUNDERS COMPANY
A Division of Elsevier Inc.

1600 John F. Kennedy Boulevard • Suite 1800 • Philadelphia, Pennsylvania 19103-2899

http://www.theclinics.com

CARDIAC ELECTROPHYSIOLOGY CLINICS Volume 2, Number 4
December 2010 ISSN 1877-9182, ISBN-13: 978-1-4557-0304-3

Editor: Barbara Cohen-Kligerman
Developmental Editor: Jessica Demetriou

Cardiac Electrophysiology Clinics (ISSN 1877-9182) is published quarterly by Elsevier Inc., 360 Park Avenue South, New York, NY 10010-1710. Months of issue are March, June, September, and December. Subscription prices are $167.00 per year for US individuals, $250.00 per year for US institutions, $88.00 per year for US students and residents, $187.00 per year for Canadian individuals, $279.00 per year for Canadian institutions, $239.00 per year for international individuals, $299.00 per year for international institutions and $126.00 per year for Canadian and foreign students/residents. To receive student/resident rate, orders must be accompanied by name of affilliated institution, date of term, and the signature of program/residency coordinator on institution letterhead. Orders will be billed at individual rate until proof of status is received. Foreign air speed delivery is included in all Clinics subscription prices. All prices are subject to change without notice. **POSTMASTER:** Send address changes to Cardiac Electrophysiology Clinics, Elsevier Health Sciences Division, Subscription Customer Service, 3251 Riverport Lane, Maryland Heights, MO 63043. **Customer Service: 1-800-654-2452 (US and Canada). From outside of the US and Canada, call 314-477-8871. Fax: 314-447-8029. E-mail: JournalsCustomerService-usa@elsevier.com (for print support); JournalsOnlineSupport-usa@elsevier.com (for online support).**

Reprints. For copies of 100 or more of articles in this publication, please contact the Commercial Reprints Department, Elsevier Inc., 360 Park Avenue South, New York, NY 10010-1710. Tel.: 212-633-3812; Fax: 212-462-1935; E-mail: reprints@elsevier.com.

Printed and bound in the United Kingdom
Transferred to Digital Print 2011

The cover illustration shows catecholaminergic, exercise-induced arrhythmias, and genetic architecture of cardiac cells.

Contributors

CONSULTING EDITORS

RANJAN K. THAKUR, MD, MPH, MBA, FHRS
Professor of Medicine and Director, Arrhythmia
Service, Thoracic and Cardiovascular Institute,
Sparrow Health System, Michigan State
University, Lansing, Michigan

ANDREA NATALE, MD, FACC, FHRS
Executive Medical Director, Texas Cardiac
Arrhythmia Institute at St David's Medical
Center, Austin, Texas; Consulting Professor,
Division of Cardiology, Stanford University,
Palo Alto, California; Clinical Associate
Professor of Medicine, Case Western Reserve
University, Cleveland, Ohio; Senior Clinical
Director, EP Services, California Pacific
Medical Center, San Francisco, California;
Department of Biomedical Engineering,
University of Texas, Austin, Texas

GUEST EDITOR

SILVIA G. PRIORI, MD, PhD
Division of Cardiology and Molecular
Cardiology, IRCCS Fondazione Salvatore
Maugeri; Department of Cardiology, University
of Pavia, Pavia, Italy; Cardiovascular Genetics
Program, Leon H. Charney Division of
Cardiology, New York University School of
Medicine, New York, New York

AUTHORS

JEFFREY B. ANDERSON, MD, MPH
Instructor of Pediatrics, The Heart Institute,
Cincinnati Children's Hospital Medical Center,
University of Cincinnati, Cincinnati, Ohio

SAMER ARNOUS, MBBS, MRCPI
Inherited Cardiovascular Disease Group,
University College London Hospitals NHS
Trust, The Heart Hospital, Westminster,
London, United Kingdom

CRISTINA BASSO, MD, PhD
Department of Medico-Diagnostic Sciences
and Special Therapies, University of Padua,
Padova, Italy

BARBARA BAUCE, MD, PhD
Department of Cardiac Thoracic and Vascular
Sciences, University of Padua Medical School,
University of Padua, Padova, Italy

D. WOODROW BENSON, MD, PhD
Professor of Pediatrics, The Heart Institute,
Cincinnati Children's Hospital Medical
Center, University of Cincinnati,
Cincinnati, Ohio

PAOLA BERNE, MD
Senior Fellow, Arrhythmia Section,
Cardiology Department, Thorax Institute,
Hospital Clínic, Institut de Investigació
Biomèdica August Pi i Sunyer (IDIBAPS),
University of Barcelona, Barcelona,
Catalonia, Spain

RAFFAELLA BLOISE, MD
Molecular Cardiology, IRCCS Fondazione
Salvatore Maugeri; Department of Cardiology,
University of Pavia, Pavia, Italy

JOSEP BRUGADA, MD, PhD
Medical Director, Arrhythmia Section,
Cardiology Department, Thorax Institute,
Hospital Clínic, Institut de Investigació
Biomèdica August Pi i Sunyer (IDIBAPS),
University of Barcelona, Barcelona,
Catalonia, Spain

MARINA CERRONE, MD
Cardiovascular Genetics Program, Leon H.
Charney Division of Cardiology, New York
University School of Medicine, New York,
New York

STÉPHANIE CHATEL, PhD
L'institut du thorax, Nantes, France

DOMENICO CORRADO, MD, PhD
Department of Cardiac Thoracic and
Vascular Sciences, University of Padua
Medical School, University of Padua,
Padova, Italy

CHRISTOPHER CRITOPH, BM
Specialist Registrar in Cardiology, The Heart
Hospital, London, United Kingdom

SAMORI CUMMINGS, MD
Cadiovascular Genetics, Leon H. Charney
Division of Cardiology, New York University
Medical Center, New York, New York

NICOLAS DERVAL, MD
Hôpital Cardiologique du Haut-Lévêque,
Université Bordeaux II, Bordeaux, France

PERRY ELLIOTT, MBBS, MD
Reader in Inherited Cardiac Disease and
Consultant Cardiologist, The Heart Hospital,
London, United Kingdom

ANDREI FORCLAZ, MD
Hôpital Cardiologique du Haut-Lévêque,
Université Bordeaux II, Bordeaux, France

STEVEN J. FOWLER, MD
Cardiovascular Genetics Program; Clinical
Cardiac Electrophysiology, Leon H. Charney
Division of Cardiology, New York University
Langone Medical Center, New York,
New York

KOJI FUKUZAWA, MD, PhD
Department of Cardiac Thoracic and Vascular
Sciences, University of Padua Medical School,
University of Padua, Padova, Italy

FIORENZO GAITA, MD
Professor, Cardiology Department, Division
of Cardiology, Cardinal Massaia Hospital,
Asti; Division of Cardiology, San Giovanni
Battista Hospital, School of Medicine,
University of Turin, Turin, Italy

ANDREW A. GRACE, MB, PhD
Research Group Head, Department of
Biochemistry, University of Cambridge;
Department of Cardiology, Papworth
Hospital, Cambridge, United Kingdom

CARLA GIUSTETTO, MD
Cardiology Department, Division of
Cardiology, Cardinal Massaia Hospital,
Asti; Division of Cardiology, San Giovanni
Battista Hospital, University of Turin,
Turin, Italy

MICHEL HAISSAGUERRE, MD
Service de Rythmologie, Hôpital Cardiologique
du Haut-Lévêque, Université Bordeaux II,
Bordeaux, France

MELEZE HOCINI, MD
Hôpital Cardiologique du Haut-Lévêque,
Université Bordeaux II, Bordeaux, France

CHRISTOPHER L-H. HUANG, PhD
Professor of Physiology, The Physiology
Department, University of Cambridge,
Downing Site, Cambridge,
United Kingdom

AMIR S. JADIDI, MD
Hôpital Cardiologique du Haut-Lévêque,
Université Bordeaux II, Bordeaux, France

PIERRE JAIS, MD
Hôpital Cardiologique du Haut-Lévêque,
Université Bordeaux II, Bordeaux, France

NICK LINTON, MD
Hôpital Cardiologique du Haut-Lévêque,
Université Bordeaux II, Bordeaux, France

XINGPENG LIU, MD
Hôpital Cardiologique du Haut-Lévêque,
Université Bordeaux II, Bordeaux, France

PHILIPPE MABO, MD
CHU Pontchaillou, Rennes, France

CLAIRE A. MARTIN, MB, BChir
Clinical Research Fellow, The Physiology Department, University of Cambridge, Cambridge, United Kingdom

ANDREA MAZZANTI, MD
Cardiology Department, Division of Cardiology, Cardinal Massaia Hospital, Asti; Division of Cardiology, San Giovanni Battista Hospital, University of Turin, Turin, Italy

WILLIAM J. MCKENNA, MD, DSc, FRCP, FESC, FACC
Inherited Cardiovascular Disease Group, University College London Hospitals NHS Trust, The Heart Hospital, Westminster; Institute of Cardiovascular Science, University College London, Camden, London, United Kingdom

FEDERICO MIGLIORE, MD
Department of Cardiac Thoracic and Vascular Sciences, University of Padua Medical School, University of Padua, Padova, Italy

SHINSUKE MIYAZAKI, MD
Hôpital Cardiologique du Haut-Lévêque, Université Bordeaux II, Bordeaux, France

NICOLA MONTEFORTE, MD
Molecular Cardiology Laboratories, Fondazione S. Maugeri IRCCS, Pavia, Italy

CARLO NAPOLITANO, MD, PhD
Molecular Cardiology Laboratories IRCCS Fondazione Salvatore Maugeri Pavia, Italy; Cadiovascular Genetics, Leon Charney Division of Cardiology, New York University Medical Center, New York, New York

VINCENT PROBST, MD, PhD
INSERM, l'institut du thorax, Nantes, France

ILARIA RIGATO, MD, PhD
Department of Cardiac Thoracic and Vascular Sciences, University of Padua Medical School, University of Padua, Padova, Italy

FRÉDÉRIC SACHER, MD
Service de Rythmologie, Hôpital Cardiologique du Haut-Lévêque, Université Bordeaux II, Bordeaux, France

DANIEL SCHERR, MD
Hôpital Cardiologique du Haut-Lévêque, Université Bordeaux II, Bordeaux, France

JEAN-JACQUES SCHOTT, PhD
L'institut du thorax, Nantes, France

SRIJITA SEN-CHOWDHRY, MRCP, MD, FESC
Inherited Cardiovascular Disease Group, Institute of Cardiovascular Science, University College London, Camden; Department of Epidemiology, Imperial College-St Mary's Campus, London, United Kingdom

ASHOK J. SHAH, MD
Hôpital Cardiologique du Haut-Lévêque, Université Bordeaux II, Bordeaux, France

PETROS SYRRIS, PhD
Inherited Cardiovascular Disease Group, Institute of Cardiovascular Science, University College London, Camden, London, United Kingdom

GAETANO THIENE, MD
Department of Medico-Diagnostic Sciences and Special Therapies, University of Padua Medical School, Padova, Italy

OLIVIER XHAET, MD
Hôpital Cardiologique du Haut-Lévêque, Université Bordeaux II, Bordeaux, France

ALESSANDRO ZORZI, MD
Department of Cardiac Thoracic and Vascular Sciences, University of Padua Medical School, University of Padua, Padova, Italy

Contents

> The sinoatrial node exhibits complex cellular and molecular structure and its proper function requires an intricate arrangement of its architecture. A better understanding of the genetic and molecular makeup of the sinoatrial node has led to improved understanding of its function as primary cardiac pacemaker and the abnormalities that may lead to sick sinus syndrome, a common clinical problem. Recently, genetic studies have begun to identify the molecular underpinnings of sick sinus syndrome. Taken together, these findings promise improved diagnosis and alternative therapies for sick sinus syndrome.

> Progressive cardiac conduction disease (PCCD), a source of considerable morbidity, comprises a heterogeneous group of conditions resulting from genetic predisposition, environmental modifiers, and other physiologic determinants, including aging. The genetic factors include numerous mutations and variants within the cardiac sodium channel gene, *SCN5A*. The electrocardiographic phenotype has variable penetrance and is associated with appearances ranging from an isolated conduction disorder to an association with tachyarrhythmias and clinically significant cardiomyopathy. A heterozygotic *Scn5a* mouse model provides evidence that PCCD may lead to cardiac remodeling consistent with clinical observations in addition to slowing of intracardiac conduction. PCCD has also been associated with the altered expression of genes encoding other proteins involved in impulse propagation, including those responsible for Ca^{2+-} activated ion channels and cytoskeletal components, both in the presence or absence of structural abnormalities.

> Catecholaminergic polymorphic ventricular tachycardia (CPVT) is an inherited arrhythmogenic disease characterized by a structurally normal heart and high lethality beginning in early childhood. The identification of its genetic bases made possible the discovery that arrhythmias are caused by intracellular calcium dysregulation. In the 9 years since the description of the genetic substrate of the disease, we have witnessed remarkable progress in the unraveling of the molecular mechanisms underlying its arrhythmogenesis. The impact of these discoveries extends beyond the field of inherited arrhythmias and sheds new light on the arrhythmogenic mechanisms in some more prevalent diseases characterized by abnormal calcium regulation, such as heart failure. Additionally, basic research studies led to the exploration

of new therapeutic strategies with potential clinical impact in the near future in reducing the still high incidence of sudden death associated with these conditions. In the current review, the authors discuss the clinical and genetic features of CPVT, highlighting pathophysiologic insights derived from experimental research and future therapeutic targets.

The Brugada syndrome is a genetically determined cardiac disorder, presenting with characteristic electrocardiogram features and high risk of sudden cardiac death from polymorphic ventricular tachycardia/ventricular fibrillation in young individuals with a structurally normal heart. Scientific knowledge about the disease has grown exponentially in recent years. Two consensus reports on the disease were published (in 2002 and 2005) in an effort to state diagnostic criteria, risk stratification, and treatment indications. However, substantial controversies remain, especially considering risk stratification of asymptomatic patients. Given the enormous amount of valuable information collected by many groups since the consensus reports, current diagnostic criteria, recommended prognostic tools, and treatment must be reviewed. This article briefly reviews recent advances in understanding of Brugada syndrome and its genetic and molecular basis, arrhythmogenic mechanisms, and clinical course. An update of tools for risk stratification and treatment of the condition is also included.

The short QT syndrome is a recently described genetic arrhythmogenic disorder, characterized by abnormally short QT intervals and a high incidence of sudden death and atrial fibrillation. Clinical manifestations may also be present in infants; a family history of cardiac sudden death is often present. Gain-of-function mutations in 3 genes encoding potassium channels and loss-of-function mutations in 2 genes encoding the cardiac L-type calcium channel have been identified. Today, the first choice therapy is implantable cardioverter-defibrillator implantation; however, pharmacologic treatment with hydroquinidine, which prolongs QT and reduces the inducibility of ventricular arrhythmias, may be proposed for children and probably for elderly asymptomatic patients.

Sudden cardiac death (SCD) is defined as an unexpected natural death from a cardiac cause within a short time period, generally less than or equal to 1 hour from the onset of symptoms, in a person without any prior condition that seems to result in instantaneous fatality. Although such a rapid death process is attributed to cardiac arrhythmia, arrhythmia often represents the final common event in a series of events precipitated by known (95%) or unknown (5%) cardiac disorder. Electrocardiographic early repolarization involving the inferolateral leads, which was labeled benign until recently, is the latest of the primary electrical cardiac diseases discovered to have significantly high prevalence in SCD cases. Careful evaluation of patients having early repolarization associated with unexplained syncope, family history of SCD, or idiopathic ventricular arrhythmias is recommended.

Arrhythmogenic Right Ventricular Cardiomyopathy

Koji Fukuzawa, Alessandro Zorzi, Federico Migliore, Ilaria Rigato, Barbara Bauce, Cristina Basso, Gaetano Thiene, and Domenico Corrado

Arrhythmogenic right ventricular cardiomyopathy (ARVC) is an inheritable heart muscle disease characterized by fibrofatty replacement of the right ventricle (RV) and by ventricular arrhythmias potentially leading to sudden cardiac death, mostly in young people and athletes. Later in the disease history, the RV becomes more diffusely involved and left ventricular involvement may result in biventricular heart failure. However, clinical diagnosis of ARVC is often difficult to make in the early stage of the disease because of the broad spectrum of phenotypic manifestations and the non-specific nature of the disease features. In 1994, an international task force proposed criteria for the clinical diagnosis of ARVC, which have been recently revised to improve their sensitivity. Causative mutations have been identified in approximately half of patients with ARVC. Advances in molecular genetics of ARVC have provided important insight into our understanding of the pathogenesis and pathophysiology of ARVC, which has contributed to the improvement of clinical management. Therapeutic strategies for the prevention of sudden death and disease progression include antiarrhythmic drugs, catheter ablation, and use of an implantable cardioverter defibrillator (ICD). ICD is the most effective tool against arrhythmic sudden death. The implantation of an ICD should be carefully evaluated because of the possibility of device/lead-related complications and inappropriate interventions. This review article focuses on the most current knowledge regarding clinical presentation, diagnosis, molecular genetics, and management strategies of ARVC.

Hypertrophic Cardiomyopathy

Christopher Critoph and Perry Elliott

Hypertrophic cardiomyopathy is a myocardial disease characterized by myocardial hypertrophy, disorganization of cardiac myocytes, and fibrosis. Twenty-five percent of patients have a dynamic left ventricular outflow tract gradient caused by the combined effects of rapid ventricular ejection, a narrowed outflow tract, and systolic anterior motion of the mitral valve. Most cases are caused by mutations in genes that encode cardiac sarcomeric proteins. Patients present at all ages with chest pain, dyspnea, palpitations, and syncope. The most important complications of the disease are sudden cardiac death, heart failure, and thromboembolism. The principal aims of management are the alleviation of symptoms and the prevention of sudden death. In patients with substantial left ventricular outflow tract obstruction, interventions that reduce the magnitude of the outflow tract gradient (disopyramide, verapamil, β-blockade, alcohol ablation of the interventricular septum, dual-chamber pacing, and surgery) often improve symptoms. Therapeutic options in patients without left ventricular outflow tract obstruction are more limited. Clinical risk stratification is used to estimate the risk of sudden death and to target effective prophylactic treatment with an implantable cardioverter defibrillator.

Genetics of Dilated Cardiomyopathy: Risk of Conduction Defects and Sudden Cardiac Death

Samer Arnous, Petros Syrris, Srijita Sen-Chowdhry, and William J. McKenna

Dilated cardiomyopathy is familial in at least 40–60% of cases and causal mutations have been identified in more than 40 different genes. Mutations in lamin A/C (LMNA) and desmosomal components appear associated with increased risk of sudden cardiac death, the latter in the context of left-dominant arrhythmogenic cardiomyopathy. Specific clinical features may be valuable in identifying patients with these mutations. Routine sequencing of all the genes implicated in dilated cardiomyopathy may not be cost-effective at present. Targeted mutation screening of LMNA and desmosomal components is recommended and may facilitate prognostication and management.

Despite the heterogeneity of substrates and clinical expressivity, genetic testing has a direct impact on clinical practice: it allows a specific diagnosis, including silent carriers (ie, asymptomatic diagnosis) and, in select diseases, the identification of a mutation has major impact for risk stratification and treatment of patients. This article addresses the role of genetic testing for each of the most epidemiologically relevant inherited arrhythmogenic diseases, specifically long QT syndrome, Brugada syndrome, catecholaminergic polymorphic ventricular tachycardia, hypertrophic cardiomyopathy, and arrhythmogenic right ventricular cardiomyopathy.

Syncope and risk of sudden death caused by ventricular tachyarrhythmia are the common manifestations of several inherited disorders. The abnormalities of the genetic makeup may directly affect proteins controlling cardiac excitability in a structurally normal heart. Other diseases manifest primarily with ventricular arrhythmias even if the genetic mutations cause structural abnormalities of the myocardium, such as arrhythmogenic right ventricular cardiomyopathy and hypertrophic cardiomyopathy. The groundbreaking discoveries that began in the 1990s and continued until the beginning of the current decade gathered fundamental knowledge about the major genes controlling cardiac excitability and conferring an increased risk of severe arrhythmias. Stemming from such knowledge is the availability of genetic diagnosis, genotype-phenotype correlation, and genotype-based risk stratification schemes. This article provides a concise description of the known genes and key mechanisms involved in the pathogenesis of inherited arrhythmias and outlines the possibilities, limitations, advantages, and potential threats of genetic testing for inherited arrhythmogenic syndromes.

Cardiac Electrophysiology Clinics

READ THE CLINICS ONLINE!

Access your subscription at:
www.theclinics.com

Foreword
From Genes to the Bedside

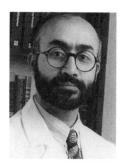
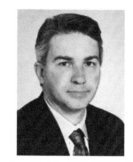

Ranjan K. Thakur, MD, MPH, MBA, FHRS   Andrea Natale, MD, FACC, FHRS
Consulting Editors

We are pleased to introduce the one-year anniversary issue of the *Cardiac Electrophysiology Clinics*, entitled "Genetics of Cardiac Arrhythmias," edited by Sylvia Priori.

All clinicians recognize that our understanding of cardiac arrhythmias has progressed beyond the "phenotype." Early on, we learned the correlation between physiology, pathology, and clinical presentation. Then, our understanding progressed to the level of the cell, correlating cellular physiology and pathology to the genesis and sustenance of cardiac arrhythmias and how to select pharmacologic agents for therapeutic effect. Although we did not fully attain the original promise of the "Sicilian Gambit," our understanding was clearly at a higher level.

While there is still much to learn at the phenotype level, as we delve deeper, our next level of understanding will be focused on elucidating the genetic bases of certain arrhythmias and the responsible molecular mechanisms. We clearly see this in our understanding of the long and short QT syndromes, the Brugada syndrome, cardiomyopathies, etc.

Dr Priori has been a leader in this field, and in this issue of the *Clinics*, she has assembled esteemed contributors who have summarized what we know today about the genetics of some common arrhythmias seen in practice. In this issue, readers will find not only food for intellectual growth, but also practical knowledge useful in day-to-day clinical practice.

One of the greatest physicists of the 20th century, Enrico Fermi, after attending a lecture, was noted to have said, "Before I came to your lecture, I was confused about the subject. Having listened to you, I am still confused, but on a higher plane." In this issue of the *Clinics*, Dr Priori and her able contributors have summarized what we know about the genetics of common clinical arrhythmias and we hope that the reader will find himself on a higher plane.

Ranjan K. Thakur, MD, MPH, MBA, FHRS
Thoracic and Cardiovascular Institute
405 West Greenlawn, Suite 400
Lansing, MI 48910, USA

Andrea Natale, MD, FACC, FHRS
Texas Cardiac Arrhythmia Institute
Center for Atrial Fibrillation at
St David's Medical Center
1015 East 32nd Street, Suite 516
Austin, TX 78705, USA

E-mail addresses:
thakur@msu.edu (R.K. Thakur)
andrea.natale@stdavids.com (A. Natale)

Card Electrophysiol Clin 2 (2010) xiii
doi:10.1016/j.ccep.2010.10.002
1877-9182/10/$ — see front matter © 2010 Elsevier Inc. All rights reserved.

Preface

How Molecular Genetics Has Reshaped Clinical Electrophysiology—From an Historical Perspective to the New Challenges

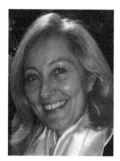

Silvia G. Priori, MD, PhD
Guest Editor

Ventricular fibrillation is most commonly encountered in the setting of structural heart disease; however, it has long been recognized that apparently healthy individuals may experience ventricular fibrillation in the absence of an overt chronic or acute cardiac disease that can justify the sudden development of such a life-threatening rhythm disturbance.

In the mid-1990s there was a surge of interest in unexplained cardiac arrest occurring in patients with a silent clinical history and a normal autopsy. The term "idiopathic ventricular fibrillation" (IVF) became a popular diagnosis for these patients. It was estimated that approximately 5 to 8% of sudden cardiac death were labeled by coroners as IVF.[1,2]

The topic attracted the interest of investigators and a registry called UCARE (Unexplained Cardiac Arrest Registry of Europe) was initiated by the European Society of Cardiology.[3] A similar initiative, the IVF-US registry, was started in North America. The two groups defined criteria to standardize the diagnosis of IVF so that a clear subset of cardiac arrest victims and survivors could be identified and thoroughly evaluated to gain more insight on this condition.[4]

As clinicians were struggling to extract from electrocardiograms, echocardiograms, and autopsies information that could shed light on IVF, a revolution was about to happen and set new paradigms in the field. It was in fact around this time that Mark Keating and his associates reported the discovery of the first genes that cause long QT syndrome,[5-7] an inherited disease diagnosed on the basis of a prolonged QT interval in patients with a structurally normal heart and high susceptibility to cardiac arrest.

At first glance, the link between IVF and the molecular basis of a rare genetic disease was rather elusive, but within a few years some unexpected findings allowed the missing link to be established. It became clear, in fact, that patients with long QT syndrome may carry a pathogenic mutation without showing an overt QT interval prolongation. These patients can appropriately be diagnosed as being affected by long QT syndrome only when genetic analysis is performed; otherwise they are likely to be defined as IVF should a cardiac arrest occur.

The presence of a disease-causing mutation in the absence of the distinguishing clinical marker of the disease in genetic terms is called

Card Electrophysiol Clin 2 (2010) xv–xvii
doi:10.1016/j.ccep.2010.11.001

"incomplete penetrance,"[8] and it turned out that it is a feature common to most channelopathies so that concealed inherited arrhythmogenic diseases represent the substrate of IVF more often than anticipated.[9]

The world of arrhythmology immediately understood the power of integrating molecular biology with clinical observations and promptly revisited some of the "unusual and unexplained diseases" in light of a genetic approach. Thanks to this innovative spirit of the electrophysiology community, collaborations with molecular biologists were promptly established and allowed the identification of the genetic basis[10,11] of diseases such as Brugada syndrome[12] and catecholaminergic polymorphic VT[13] associated with increased risk of sudden death in patients showing a completely unremarkable ECG.

In the early 1990s the world of cardiomyopathies experienced a similar "revolution" as diseases called "idiopathic" in old cardiology textbooks, such as hypertrophic cardiomyopathy or nonischemic dilated cardiomyopathy, were recognized as familial diseases and their genetic substrates started being discovered.[14,15] These findings also impacted clinical electrophysiology given that arrhythmic death is a frequent adverse outcome in patients with cardiomyopathies.

In less than two decades the field of molecular cardiology exploded: as of today a division of molecular cardiology is present in many clinical and academic cardiology centers worldwide and electrophysiology fellows appropriately search for programs that include training on the genetic basis of arrhythmias. This innovative area of electrophysiology is bringing new challenges and new opportunities.

Often the expertise required to interpret results of genetic testing needs the partnership of the clinical electrophysiologist and the cardio-geneticist: a new professional figure that combines competence in arrhythmia management and deep knowledge of the molecular substrates of channelopathies and cardiomyopathies.

Clinical electrophysiologists are called to learn when and why genetic testing should be requested for their patients. They should become able to define when genetic counseling is essential to communicate complex genetic results to patients or when dealing with delicate issues such as prenatal diagnosis. They should also become aware that, in some instances, the specific mutation or the gene in which a mutation is found may bear important implications for risk stratification and management of their patients. All of these aspects provide an opportunity for advancing the field, and by facilitating interactions between clinical electrophysiologists and cardio-geneticists they eventually will facilitate discovery of novel gene-targeted therapies for patients. They, however, pose challenges as collaboration between "genetics" and "electrophysiology" requires time and efforts to fill knowledge gaps on both sides.

In order to contribute to cross-fertilization between geneticists and clinicians we have provided in this issue an updated overview of inherited arrhythmogenic syndromes with a focus on the practical impact of the applications of genetic analysis to patient management. With this goal in mind, leading experts in the field have been invited to contribute to this volume that I do hope will be useful to experienced electrophysiologists and to fellows in training as well, to help them master the fundamental advancement in genetics of cardiac arrhythmias. In this issue we are covering the major inherited arrhythmogenic syndromes with the exception of long QT syndrome, which we will extensively address in a future dedicated volume.

Silvia G. Priori, MD, PhD
Division of Cardiology and Molecular Cardiology
IRCCS Fondazione Salvatore Maugeri
Pavia, Italy

Department of Cardiology
University of Pavia
Pavia, Italy

Cardiovascular Genetics Program
Leon H. Charney Division of Cardiology
New York University School of Medicine
New York, New York, USA

E-mail addresses:
silvia.priori@nyumc.org
silvia.priori@fsm.it

REFERENCES

1. Poole JE, Bardy GH. Sudden cardiac death. In: Zipes DP, Jalife J, editors. Cardiac electrophysiology. From cell to bedside, Philadelphia (PA): W.B. Saunders; 1995. p. 812–32.

2. Behr ER, Casey A, Sheppard M, et al. Sudden arrhythmic death syndrome: a national survey of sudden unexplained cardiac death. Heart 2007;93: 601–5.

3. Priori SG, Borggrefe M, Camm AJ, et al. Unexplained cardiac arrest: the need of a prospective registry. Eur Heart J 1992;13:1445–6.

4. Survivors of out-of-hospital cardiac arrest with apparently normal heart need for definition and standardized clinical evaluation. Consensus Statement

of the Joint Steering Committees of the Unexplained Cardiac Arrest Registry of Europe and of the Idiopathic Ventricular Fibrillation Registry of the United States. Circulation 1997;95:265–72.

5. Wang Q, Shen J, Splawski I, et al. SCN5A mutations associated with an inherited cardiac arrhythmia, long QT syndrome. Cell 1995;80:805–11.

6. Curran ME, Splawski I, Timothy KW, et al. A molecular basis for cardiac arrhythmia: HERG mutations cause long QT syndrome. Cell 1995;80:795–803.

7. Wang Q, Curran ME, Splawski I, et al. Positional cloning of a novel potassium channel gene: KVLQT1 mutations cause cardiac arrhythmias. Nat Genet 1996;12:17–23.

8. Priori SG, Napolitano C, Schwartz PJ. Low penetrance in the long-QT syndrome: clinical impact. Circulation 1999;99:529–33.

9. Priori SG, Napolitano C, Grillo M. Concealed arrhythmogenic syndromes: the hidden substrate of idiopathic ventricular fibrillation? Cardiovasc Res 2001; 50:218–23.

10. Wang DW, Yazawa K, George AL, et al. Characterization of human cardiac Na+ channel mutations in the congenital long QT syndrome. Proc Natl Acad Sci U S A 1996;93:13200–5.

11. Priori SG, Napolitano C, Tiso N, et al. Mutations in the cardiac ryanodine receptor gene (hRyR2) underlie catecholaminergic polymorphic ventricular tachycardia. Circulation 2000;102:r49–53.

12. Brugada P, Brugada J. Right bundle branch block, persistent ST segment elevation and sudden cardiac death: a distinct clinical and electrocardiographic syndrome. A multicenter report. J Am Coll Cardiol 1992; 20:1391–6.

13. Coumel P, Fidelle J, Lucet V, et al. Catecholamine-induced severe ventricular arrhythmias with Adams-Stokes syndrome in children: report of four cases. Br Heart J 1978;40(suppl):28–37.

14. Geisterfer-Lowrance AA, Kass S, Tanigawa G, et al. A molecular basis for familial hypertrophic cardiomyopathy: a beta cardiac myosin heavy chain gene missense mutation. Cell 1990;62: 999–1006.

15. Burkett EL, Hershberger RE. Clinical and genetic issues in familial dilated cardiomyopathy. J Am Coll Cardiol 2005;45:969–81.

Genetics of Sick Sinus Syndrome

Jeffrey B. Anderson, MD, MPH,
D. Woodrow Benson, MD, PhD*

KEYWORDS

- Sick sinus syndrome • Sinus node • SCN5A
- HCN • Connexins

Sick sinus syndrome (SSS) was first described over four decades ago as a complicating arrhythmia following cardioversion,[1] and shortly thereafter its electrocardiographic features were defined.[2] The disorder is characterized by persistent inappropriate sinus bradycardia, episodes of sinoatrial (SA) block, or chronotropic incompetence.[3] Episodes of atrial tachycardia coexisting with sinus bradycardia (tachycardia-bradycardia syndrome) are also common in this disorder (**Fig. 1**).[4] Despite extensive efforts to better understand the mechanism of SSS in terms of abnormal automaticity, sinus node exit block, or impaired intraatrial conduction and excitability, this has remained largely an electrocardiographic diagnosis.[4]

The SA node is a complex structure and its proper function requires an intricate arrangement of cellular and molecular components. SSS, a misnomer, once thought to be simply a problem with the automaticity initiated within the SA node, can be secondary to a number of different molecular, cellular, and structural abnormalities. For example, the SA node core, where automaticity arises, may be working properly with abnormal conduction from the SA node to the remainder of the atrium. As discussed later in this article, patients diagnosed with SSS may have problems with automaticity, propagation of electrical impulses from the SA node to the remainder of the heart, abnormalities related to autonomic influences on the SA node, or a combination of these problems. SSS may occur in the absence of structural heart disease, but "atrial disease" is a recurring theme whether in the elderly with acquired heart

disease or in young survivors of congenital heart disease surgery. Patients of any age with SSS may exhibit varied symptoms including presyncope or syncope and activity intolerance, and SSS may even be the cause of sudden cardiac arrest. The course of SSS can be intermittent and unpredictable, related to the severity of the underlying heart disease. Although SSS is more common in the elderly and in those with structural heart disease, its true incidence is unknown because the features of SSS have not been evaluated in the general population in a standardized manner.[3]

SINUS NODE ARCHITECTURE AND PHYSIOLOGY
Gross and Microscopic Anatomy

Keith and Flack[5] first described the SA node in 1907. Of their findings they wrote, "There is a remarkable remnant of primitive fibers persisting at the sinoauricular junction in all the mammalian hearts examined… in them the dominating rhythm of the heart is believed to normally arise."[5] The anatomic and histologic structure of the SA node is conserved across vertebrates.[5] The SA node is a right atrial structure that is subepicardial and can be located at the junction of the crista terminalis (CT) at the superior cavoatrial junction.[6] It is shaped like a flattened ellipse and the prominent SA nodal artery passes through its body. Multiple autonomic nerves course to both its poles.[7] The SA node is an extensive structure, encompassing tissue from the superior to the inferior vena cava[8] and the size and tissue thickness of the SA node

No external funding was used for this manuscript. The authors have no financial relationships to disclose.
The Heart Institute, Cincinnati Children's Hospital Medical Center, University of Cincinnati, 3333 Burnet Avenue, ML 7042, Cincinnati, OH 45229, USA
* Corresponding author.
E-mail address: woody.benson@cchmc.org

Card Electrophysiol Clin 2 (2010) 499–507
doi:10.1016/j.ccep.2010.09.001

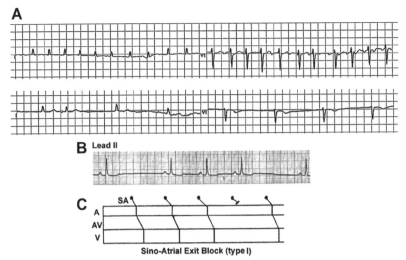

Fig. 1. Electrocardiographic findings in sick sinus syndrome. (*A*) Tachycardia-bradycardia. (*Courtesy of* Michael Laurent, MD, Department of Internal Medicine, University Hospital Leuven, Leuven, Belgium.) (*B*) Atrial fibrillation. (*Courtesy of* Michael Laurent, MD, Department of Internal Medicine, University Hospital Leuven, Leuven, Belgium.) (*C*) Sinoatrial block. (*Courtesy of* Frank Yanowitz, Salt Lake City, UT.)

varies between species.[6] In humans, the SA node lies beneath the epicardial surface with a layer of atrial muscle between the SA node and the endocardium.[9] This layer of atrial muscle, along with connective tissue in the region of the SA node, is thought to protect the area against high wall stresses.[10] Microscopically, the SA node is characterized by a complex pattern of cells within a fibrous stroma. Near its periphery there is an outer coat of working atrial myocytes. The function of the specialized cells of the SA node is conduction rather than contraction; therefore, they are smaller, have fewer contractile elements, and expend less energy than surrounding myocytes (**Fig. 2**).[7]

Molecular Architecture

The molecular organization of the SA node is complex but serves as a template to understand the characteristics that allow for its role as the primary pacemaker in the heart.[11,12] **Fig. 3** shows a section cut through the SA node. SA node tissue arises from the intercaval region and persists to the endocardial surface near the CT and overlaps the atrial muscle. In the atrial muscle, Cx43 is expressed and Cx45 is absent. In contrast, in the SA node core, Cx43 is absent and Cx45 is expressed, whereas in the periphery of the SA node, both Cx43 and Cx45 are expressed. Atrial muscle expresses atrial natriuretic peptide (ANP) but not neurofilament, and the SA node core and periphery express neurofilament but not ANP. Neurofilament is a cytoskeletal protein found in nerve cells.

Because it is expressed in the SA node and other cardiac pacemaker and conducting tissues but not in the rest of the heart, it has been suggested that these tissues are neural in origin.[13] On the basis of these markers, three cell types can be identified: (1) ANP-negative/neurofilament-positive/Cx43-negative/Cx45-positive central cells, (2) ANP-negative/neurofilament-positive/Cx43-positive/Cx45-positive peripheral cells, and (3) ANP-positive/neurofilament-negative/Cx43-positive/Cx45-negative atrial cells. It is important to minimize electrotonic coupling.[14]

Gap junctions and connexins

Electron microscopy has demonstrated the presence of gap junctions in the SA node and in other myocardial tissue. Gap junctions are made up of serially linked channels (connexons) contributed to by two opposing cell membranes. These junctions allow for the passage of small molecules (<1 kDa) between two adjacent cells.[10] Each connexon is composed of six transmembrane proteins called "connexins." In cardiac tissue, three main connexin isoforms are found: (1) Cx40, (2) Cx43, and (3) Cx45.[14] A fourth connexin, Cx30.2, has been identified in murine conduction tissue; its human ortholog is Cx31.9.[14] There is regional and tissue-specific expression of different connexin isoforms within the heart (**Fig. 4**). Cx40 is mainly expressed in the atrial myocytes, the AV node, His-bundle, and the ventricular conduction system. Cx43 is expressed in atrial and ventricular myocytes and within the distal portions of the ventricular conduction system. Cx43 is also

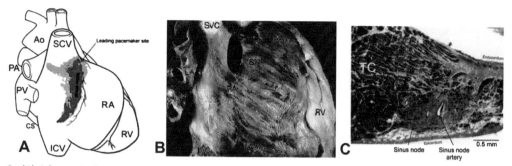

Fig. 2. (*A*) Schematic diagram of dorsal view of rabbit heart showing location and extent of central (*red*) and peripheral (*blue*) sinus node tissue. (*From* Dobrzynski H, Boyett MR, Anderson RH. New insights into pacemaker activity: promoting understanding of sick sinus syndrome. Circulation 2007;115(14):1921–32; with permission.) (*B*) The sinus node lies subepicardially in the terminal groove of the right atrium (*right lateral view*). (*From* Edwards W. Cardiac anatomy and examination of cardiac specimens. In: Allen HD, Driscoll DJ, Shaddy RE, et al, editors. Moss and Adams heart disease in infants, children, and adolescents, Vol. 1. 7th edition. Philadelphia: Lippincott Williams and Wilkins; 2008. p. 2–33; with permission.) (*C*) Masson's trichrome-stained section through human sinus node. (*From* Dobrzynski H, Boyett MR, Anderson RH. New insights into pacemaker activity: promoting understanding of sick sinus syndrome. Circulation 2007;115(14):1921–32; with permission.)

expressed in SA node periphery but not at its core.[10] There is localization of Cx45 in the SA node, the AV node, His bundle, and bundle branches. Although the structures of connexin isoforms are similar, the biophysical properties of the channels they form are very different.[15,16] For example, gap junction conductance follows the sequence of Cx40>Cx43>Cx45>Cx30.2/Cx31.9 consistent with better conductance in atrial tissue compared with that at the SA node core.[17] The differences in electrical properties of gap junctions help explain regional differences in electrical conduction. In addition, there are regional differences in the total number of gap junctions participating in cellular communication. Gap junctions are sparsely found in the SA node and seen in great quantity in atrial tissue.[18]

Gap junctions in the SA node play a role in both automaticity and transfer of electrical impulses to the surrounding myocardium.[19] At the SA node core Cx45 is the predominant connexin in gap junction proteins.[20] There are few total gap

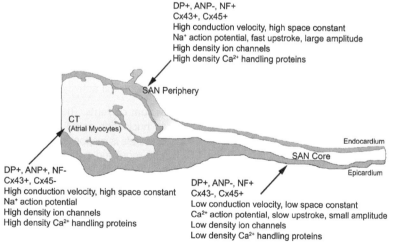

Fig. 3. Schematic diagram illustrating molecular architecture of the SA node. The anatomic section is through the crista terminalis (CT) and intercaval region of rabbit showing the relative relation of CT with SA node periphery and SA node core. The distribution of cell types expressing (+ve, positive) or not expressing (−ve, negative) the indicated molecular components is depicted. The section is oriented so that endocardium is up and epicardium is on the lower side. The green area depicts adipocytes and other connective tissue surrounding the SA node region. (*Modified from* Boyett MR, Dobrzynski H, Lancaster MK, et al. Sophisticated architecture is required for the sinoatrial node to perform its normal pacemaker function. J Cardiovasc Electrophysiol 2003;14(1): 104–6; with permission.)

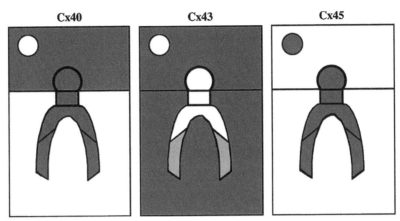

Fig. 4. Chamber-specific expression of Cx40, Cx43, and Cx45 in the mouse heart. (*From* Jansen JA, van Veen TA, de Bakker JM, et al. Cardiac connexins and impulse propagation. J Mol Cell Cardiol 2010;48(1):76–82;with permission.)

junctions found at the SA node core,[18] where little coupling is necessary for synchronization of electrical impulses of individual cells.[21] In the periphery of the SA node Cx40 and Cx43 are both expressed. Studies in mice using knock-out models of Cx43 and Cx45 demonstrated no significant heart rate abnormalities, but Cx40$^{-/-}$ mice did display breakthrough activation of pacemaker activity at locations distant from the SA node, as seen in wild-type mice.[22] Haploinsufficiency or deletion of Cx43 has also been shown to have no effect on SA nodal function.[23] The fact that the SA node seems to function well, even with reduced expression or absence of apparently essential connexins, supports the thought that little coupling is needed for electrical propagation within the SA node itself.[14]

Connexins play an important role in electrical propagation through atrial tissue. Murine models haploinsufficient or deficient for Cx43 show no changes in electrical impulse propagation through the atria.[24] There have been mixed results in studies of Cx40 knock-out mice and the effect on atrial electrical impulse propagation.[25,26] Although the deficiency of Cx40 or Cx43 expression may not itself lead to decreased atrial electrical propagation, there does seem to be a relationship between impulse propagation velocity and the ratio of atrial Cx40 and Cx43 expression.[27,28]

Ion channels, handling proteins, and receptors
Sodium and calcium current The inward sodium current (I_{Na}) is responsible for the initial upstroke of the action potential within atrial myocardium. Within the SA node core there is an absence of I_{Na}, resulting in a slow initial upstroke of the action potential.[29] Blockade of I_{Na} with tetradotoxin, in

the rabbit, results in no effect on electrical activity recorded from the SA node core.[30] The cardiac isoform of the channel responsible for I_{Na} is most abundantly expressed in atrial muscle and has been shown to be expressed in lower amounts within the SA node and to be absent from the SA node core in a murine model.[31]

Two separate inward Ca^{2+} currents have been identified in SA node core tissue. A long-lasting current (I_{CaL}) and a transient current (I_{CaT}) serve separate roles in action potential formation. I_{CaL} is the main contributor to the initial upstroke of the action potential in the SA node core and also plays a role in the plateau portion of the action potential. $Ca_v1.2$ is the principle isoform responsible for I_{CaL} in atrial myocardial tissue. In the SA node, however, $Ca_v1.3$ is the principle isoform.[32] I_{CaT} contributes to the last two thirds of the diastolic depolarization. Blockage of both calcium currents has been shown to suppress spontaneous electrical activity in the SA node core.[30,33]

Potassium currents The hyperpolarization-activated cyclic nucleotide-gated (HCN) family (HCN1–4) of ion channels is responsible for I_f. These channels are directly regulated by cyclic adenosine monophosphate (cAMP).[34] This current is inward in direction and carries both Na and K ions. I_f increases when cellular cAMP levels are elevated during sympathetic stimulation and decreases when levels are reduced during vagal stimulation.[35] Further evidence of the contribution of I_f to automaticity has been documented in observation of a decrease in automaticity in both humans and rodents when I_f is specifically blocked with the selective I_f inhibitor ivabradine.[36–38] Two of the four known genes encoding HCN channel subunits, HCN2 and HCN4, are predominantly expressed in the heart.[39] The most abundant isoform of this channel within the SA node is HCN4, and

HCN4 is more abundant within the SA node than in the atrial myocardium. Human genetic[40] and pharmacologic[36,41] studies have suggested a significant role for HCN4 subunits in SA nodal pacemaking in humans and rodents. However, targeted deletions of HCN4 in adult mice were found to cause sinus pauses but to have no effect on heart rate regulation.[42] Similar observations were made in adult heterozygous knock-in mice expressing a cAMP binding–deficient HCN4 subunit.[43]

Besides the HCN family, there are several potassium currents that are important in SA nodal function. The transient outward potassium current (I_{to}) activates and inactivates quickly and is responsible for the initial phase of repolarization and, in part, determines the duration of the action potential.[8] In the rabbit, I_{to} has been shown to be present at a higher density in the SA node than in atrial myocardium.[10] Delayed-rectifier potassium currents are also important in determining the duration of the action potential initiated in the SA node. During SA nodal action potential formation there are rapid and slow delayed rectifier potassium currents (I_{Kr}) and (I_{Ks}). Both help to further repolarization and determine maximum diastolic potential.[44] The inward rectifier potassium current ($I_{K,1}$) participates in stabilization of the resting potential in myocardium. The maximum diastolic potential of the sinus node is significantly more electrically positive than that of the surrounding atrial tissue. Several isotypes of the inward rectifier potassium channel are present in myocardial tissue. $K_{V1.4}$ is primarily found in atrial myocardium and KV4.2 is primarily found in sinus nodal tissue.[32]

Calcium handling proteins There are several proteins involved with calcium movement within SA node and atrial tissue. The arrival of the action potential leads to an increase in cytoplasmic Ca brought about by and influx of extracellular Ca. This Ca influx triggers a further release of calcium-mediated calcium release from the sarcoplasmic reticulum (SR) by way of the ryanodine receptor.[8] The cardiac ryanodine receptor mRNA and protein are expressed within the SA node core but is more abundant in the periphery of the SA node and in atrial tissue.[45] Once the membrane begins to repolarize Ca begins to be removed from the cytosol back to the SR by means of the SR Ca pump, SERCA2a.[8] SERCA2a is present within the SA node core but more abundantly in the periphery of the SA node and in atrial tissue.[45] Although most Ca release from the SR occurs during action potential formation (depolarization) there is some slow Ca release from the SR during diastolic repolarization. Within the SA node core

this occurs as a result of high cAMP levels.[44] The release of Ca from the SR during diastolic depolarization activates a Na/Ca exchanger (NCX), which results in an inward current that contributes to depolarization. Three isoforms of the NCX have been identified (NXC1–NCX3),[8] but only NCX1 has been identified in pacemaking cells from several animals and is present in equal concentration within the SA node and atrial tissue.[45] If intracellular stores of Ca are depleted, the influx of extracellular Ca can be augmented by transient receptor potential canonical channels. These channels have been identified in the SA node in the mouse and may be involved in pacemaking.[46]

Receptors Adenosine, adrenergic, and muscarinic receptors are all present in SA nodal tissue. Adrenergic $\alpha1a$, $\alpha2a$, $\alpha2b$, and $\alpha3$ adenosine receptors have all been identified. The α_1 and α_2 adrenergic receptors are all detectable at varying levels within the SA node. Of the muscarinic receptors, M2 are present in SA nodal tissue and M1 receptors have not been detected.[45] The presence of these receptors within the SA node gives some evidence as to the pharmacologic mechanism of action on the SA node of these classes of medications.

Physiology

The SA node is the physiologic pacemaker in the human heart and is predominantly responsible for autonomous heartbeat generation. The complex mechanisms underlying SA nodal automaticity remain incompletely understood. However, heart rate control is regulated through control of SA nodal automaticity by the autonomic nervous system; cholinergic stimulation slows spontaneous SA nodal activity and β-adrenergic stimulation accelerates spontaneous SA nodal activity.[47]

The action potential, initiated in the SA node core, propagates first into the SA node periphery and then into the surrounding atrial tissue. The speed of action potential propagation increases as distance from the SA node core increases. After electrical impulse propagation, there is stable resting electrical potential in the atrial myocardium. In the SA node, however, the tissue is more depolarized and there is further time–dependent depolarization, leading to initiation of the next action potential on reaching threshold. There is minimization of electronic coupling between the SA node and the surrounding atrial tissue. Although there is no distinct border between the SA node and the surrounding atrial tissue, the periphery of the SA node is surrounded by a layer of connective tissue. There is also poor electrical conduction velocity in the SA node core compared with conduction velocity in atrial tissue. These two properties act to protect the SA node from electrical activity in the atrium that may suppress its pacemaking functions.[48]

GENETIC ORIGINS OF SSS

From this discussion of the complex molecular makeup of the SA node, SSS may result from a number of genetic abnormalities leading to mutations in proteins important for its function. Family clustering of SSS has been reported and both autosomal–recessive (MIM #608567) and autosomal–dominant (MIM #163800) forms have been described. However, to date only a few examples have been identified.

HCN ion channels are important in the automaticity of the SA node core. HCN4 mutations have been identified in two studies of patients with SSS manifesting as marked sinus bradycardia and chronotropic incompetence.[40,49] Using HCN4 as a candidate gene, both studies identified a heterozygous 1-bp deletion (1631delC) in axon 5 of the human HCN4 gene. The mutant (HCN4-573X) is predicted to have a truncated C-terminus and lack the cyclic nucleotide–binding domain. COS-7 cells transiently transected with HCN4-573X coda exhibited normal intracellular trafficking and membrane integration of HCN4-573X subunits. However, patch-clamp experiments showed that HCN4-573X channels mediated If-like currents that were insensitive to increased cellular cAMP levels. Co-expression experiments identified a dominant–negative effect of HCN4-573X subunits on wild-type subunits. Together, these data indicate that the cardiac If channels are functionally expressed but with altered biophysical properties. To study the pathogenesis of HCN4-573X, Alig and colleagues[43] generated mice with heart-specific and inducible expression of a human HCN4-mutation (573X). They found that conditional expression of the mutation causes elimination of the cAMP sensitivity of If and decreases the maximum firing rates of SAN pacemaker cells. In conscious mice, hHCN4-573X expression leads to a marked reduction in heart rate at rest and during exercise. Despite the complete loss of camp sensitivity of If, the relative extent of SAN cell frequency and heart rate regulation are preserved. These results demonstrate that cAMP-mediated regulation of If determines basal and maximal heart rates but does not play an indispensable role in heart rate adaptation during physical activity.

Sodium channels are essential for orderly progression of action potentials from the SA node core, through its periphery, and to the surrounding atrial tissue. Abnormalities in the genes coding for sodium channels have been examined in families with SSS. Inherited abnormalities in the alpha-subunit of I_{Na} are associated with three distinct channelopathies: (1) congenital long QT syndrome,[50] (2) idiopathic ventricular fibrillation,[50,51] and (3) progressive cardiac conduction system disease.[52,53] Recent reports of mutational analyses have revealed more than 200 distinct mutations in SCN5A, of which at least 20 mutations are associated with SSS.[54] In addition to this variable expressivity, heterozygous SCN5A mutations have also shown incomplete penetrance. Compound heterozygous SCN5A mutations have also been shown to be associated with a recessive form of congenital SSS.[4] Benson and colleagues[4] identified individuals with SSS characterized by sinus bradycardia and loss of atrial excitability (atrial standstill). Compound heterozygous nucleotide changes in SCN5A were identified in five individuals from three kindreds who carried the diagnosis of SSS. Because SCN5A is not expressed in the SA node and SA node action potentials are not dependent on SCN5A, primary dysfunction of the SA node seems unlikely. However, because SA node dysfunction caused by failure of impulses to conduct into adjacent atrial myocardium (exit block) has been suggested as a cause of SSS,[43,44] it has been speculated that this is a plausible mechanism to explain this SCN5A-linked disorder.

In addition, certain genetic variants of Cx40 with accompanying SCN5A mutations have been shown to result in the atrial standstill phenotype.[55] Groenewegen and colleagues[56] studied a large family with atrial standstill. They identified heterozygosity for a mutation in SCN5A, a G→A substitution in the first nucleotide of codon 1275 leading to the substitution of Asp by Asn (D1275 N). Each family member affected by atrial standstill shared this haplotype; however, this mutation also was identified in some unaffected relatives. In addition, direct sequencing of the coding region of the Cx40 gene revealed changes in the proximal promoter: a G→A change at 44 nucleotides upstream of the transcription start site, and an A→G change in exon 1 at 71 nucleotides downstream of the transcription start site. Genotyping of all relatives revealed homozygosity for these base changes in all affected individuals and in unaffected relatives. Although mutations in both SCN5A and Cx40 were seen in affected and unaffected individuals, the occurrence of the SCN5a-D1275 N mutation and the rare Cx40 genotypes were only seen in the individuals with atrial standstill and in none of the unaffected relatives.[56] By themselves, the effect of each mutation is sufficient to result in the rare phenotype of atrial standstill. The mutation in SCN5A interferes with electrical impulse generation and the mutation in Cx40 leads to impairment of propagation of any electrical activity.[56]

MOLECULAR BIOPACEMAKER

SSS can result in various clinical symptoms including presyncope or syncope, chronotropic incompetence, or significant sinus bradycardia or sinus tachycardia that cause activity intolerance or even sudden death. The current treatment options for sinus node dysfunction include medical management to control tachyarrythmias and implanted pacemakers to counter bradyarrhythmia or sinus arrest. Implanted pacemakers are well tolerated but do require invasive placement and have a limited generator life, leading to multiple invasive procedures for replacement if needed at a young age. In the postgenomic era, there has been some interest in alternative molecular therapies for individuals with SSS.

The SA node is highly adapted to its role as the primary pacemaker. Its mix of ionic currents fits it for the pacemaking function, but in addition its poor electrical coupling protects it from the inhibitory hyperpolarizing influence of the surrounding atrial tissue. Studies to date indicate the challenges to developing a biopacemaker. Several groups over the past several years have explored the possibility of a biologic pacemaker that would ultimately replace implanted pacemakers. Proposed strategies include gene therapy, transplantation of donor excitable myocardium, and the delivery of modified embryonic stem cells to the heart. Fetal and neonatal cardiac cells have been shown to functionally integrate and act as an ectopic pacemaker when transplanted into the myocardium of dogs, pigs, and guinea pigs.[57,58] Gene therapy approaches that have been discussed include overexpression of β-adrenergic receptors; suppression of the potassium inward-rectifier current, I_{K1}; and inserting the pacemaker gene, HCN2, into the atrium using adenoviral or naked plasma vectors.[59] Another approach in the biologic treatment of SA node dysfunction is the possibility of engraftment of embryonic stem cells that have been differentiated into cardiac myocytes, into atrial tissue.[60]

Although each of these biologic approaches have shown some promise in addressing the problem of SSS they each address specific parts of a complex system. The intricacy of the anatomic and molecular design of the SA node allows for its function as the primary pacemaker of the heart. This complex design includes not only the differences in cellular makeup compared with surrounding atrial tissue but also differences in cellular makeup within the SA node itself. Each part of the SA node, at a cellular and subcellular level, plays an individual role in the initiation and propagation of electrical impulses that create normal electrical physiology within the heart. Addressing one piece of this complex puzzle is a start to creating a solution for SA node dysfunction, but a complete solution needs to include a group of interventions that create a similar configuration to the SA node.

SUMMARY

The SA node exhibits complex cellular and molecular structure and its proper function requires an intricate arrangement of its architecture. A better understanding of the genetic and molecular makeup of the SA node has led to improved understanding of its function as primary cardiac pacemaker and the abnormalities that may lead to SSS, a common clinical problem. Recently, genetic studies have begun to identify the molecular underpinnings of SSS. Taken together, these findings promise improved diagnosis and alternative therapies for SSS.

REFERENCES

1. Lown B. Electrical reversion of cardiac arrhythmias. Br Heart J 1967;29(4):469–89.
2. Ferrer MI. The sick sinus syndrome in atrial disease. JAMA 1968;206(3):645–6.
3. Brignole M. Sick sinus syndrome. Clin Geriatr Med 2002;18(2):211–27.
4. Benson DW, Wang DW, Dyment M, et al. Congenital sick sinus syndrome caused by recessive mutations in the cardiac sodium channel gene (SCN5A). J Clin Invest 2003;112(7):1019–28.
5. Keith A, Flack M. The form and nature of the muscular connections between the primary divisions of the vertebrate heart. J Anat Physiol 1907;41(Pt 3): 172–89.
6. Opthof T. The mammalian sinoatrial node. Cardiovasc Drugs Ther 1988;1(6):573–97.
7. Edwards W. Cardiac anatomy and examination of cardiac specimens. In: Allen HD, Driscoll DJ, Shaddy RE, et al, editors. Moss and Adams heart disease in infants, children, and adolescents, vol. 1. 7th edition. Philadelphia: Lippincott Williams and Wilkins; 2008. p. 2–33.
8. Boyett MR, Tellez J, Dobrzynski H. The sinoatrial node: its complex structure and unique ion channel gene program. In: Zipes, Jalife J, editors. Cardiac electrophysiology: from cell to bedside, vol. 5. Philadelphia: W.B. Saunders; 2009. p. 127–38.

9. Anderson RH, Becker AE. Anatomy of the conduction tissues and accessory atrioventricular connections. In: Zipes DP, Jalife J, editors. Cardiac
electrophysiology from cell to bedside. Philadelphia:
W.B. Saunders; 1990. p. 240–8.

10. Boyett MR, Honjo H, Kodama I. The sinoatrial node,
a heterogeneous pacemaker structure. Cardiovasc
Res 2000;47(4):658–87.

11. Dobrzynski H, Li J, Tellez J, et al. Computer three-
dimensional reconstruction of the sinoatrial node.
Circulation 2005;111(7):846–54.

12. Wittwer M, Fluck M, Hoppeler H, et al. Prolonged un-
loading of rat soleus muscle causes distinct adapta-
tions of the gene profile. FASEB J 2002;16(8):884–6.

13. Vitadello M, Colpo P, Gorza L. Rabbit cardiac and
skeletal myocytes differ in constitutive and inducible
expression of the glucose-regulated protein GRP94.
Biochem J 1998;332(Pt 2):351–9.

14. Jansen JA, van Veen TA, de Bakker JM, et al.
Cardiac connexins and impulse propagation. J Mol
Cell Cardiol 2010;48(1):76–82.

15. Saez JC, Berthoud VM, Branes MC, et al. Plasma
membrane channels formed by connexins: their
regulation and functions. Physiol Rev 2003;83(4):
1359–400.

16. van Veen AA, van Rijen HV, Opthof T. Cardiac gap junction channels: modulation of expression and channel
properties. Cardiovasc Res 2001;51(2):217–29.

17. Weingart R. Biophysical properties of gap junctions.
In: Zipes, Jalife J, editors. Cardiac electrophysi-
ology: from cell to bedside, vol. 5. Philadelphia:
W.B. Saunders; 2009. p. 149–55.

18. Saffitz JE, Green KG, Schuessler RB. Structural determinants of slow conduction in the canine sinus node.
J Cardiovasc Electrophysiol 1997;8(7):738–44.

19. Jongsma HJ. Diversity of gap junctional proteins:
does it play a role in cardiac excitation? J Cardiovasc
Electrophysiol 2000;11(2):228–30.

20. Davis LM, Rodefeld ME, Green K, et al. Gap junction
protein phenotypes of the human heart and conduction
system. J Cardiovasc Electrophysiol 1995;6(10 Pt 1):
813–22.

21. Wilders R, Verheijck EE, Kumar R, et al. Model
clamp and its application to synchronization of
rabbit sinoatrial node cells. Am J Physiol 1996;
271(5 Pt 2):H2168–82.

22. Bagwe S, Berenfeld O, Vaidya D, et al. Altered
right atrial excitation and propagation in connex-
in40 knockout mice. Circulation 2005;112(15):
2245–53.

23. Eckardt D, Theis M, Degen J, et al. Functional role of
connexin43 gap junction channels in adult mouse
heart assessed by inducible gene deletion. J Mol
Cell Cardiol 2004;36(1):101–10.

24. Thomas SA, Schuessler RB, Berul CI, et al. Dispa-
rate effects of deficient expression of connexin43
on atrial and ventricular conduction: evidence for

chamber-specific molecular determinants of
conduction. Circulation 1998;97(7):686–91.

25. VanderBrink BA, Sellitto C, Saba S, et al. Connex-
in40-deficient mice exhibit atrioventricular nodal
and infra-Hisian conduction abnormalities.
J Cardiovasc Electrophysiol 2000;11(11):1270–6.

26. Verheule S, van Batenburg CA, Coenjaerts FE, et al.
Cardiac conduction abnormalities in mice lacking
the gap junction protein connexin40. J Cardiovasc
Electrophysiol 1999;10(10):1380–9.

27. Beauchamp P, Yamada KA, Baertschi AJ, et al.
Relative contributions of connexins 40 and 43 to
atrial impulse propagation in synthetic strands of
neonatal and fetal murine cardiomyocytes. Circ
Res 2006;99(11):1216–24.

28. Kanagaratnam P, Rothery S, Patel P, et al. Relative
expression of immunolocalized connexins 40 and
43 correlates with human atrial conduction properties. J Am Coll Cardiol 2002;39(1):116–23.

29. Honjo H, Boyett MR, Kodama I, et al. Correlation
between electrical activity and the size of rabbit sinoatrial node cells. J Physiol 1996;496(Pt 3):795–808.

30. Kodama I, Nikmaram MR, Boyett MR, et al. Regional
differences in the role of the Ca2+ and Na+
currents in pacemaker activity in the sinoatrial
node. Am J Physiol 1997;272(6 Pt 2):H2793–806.

31. Lei M, Jones SA, Liu J, et al. Requirement of
neuronal- and cardiac-type sodium channels for
murine sinoatrial node pacemaking. J Physiol
2004;559(Pt 3):835–48.

32. Tellez JO, Dobrzynski H, Greener ID, et al. Differential expression of ion channel transcripts in atrial
muscle and sinoatrial node in rabbit. Circ Res
2006;99(12):1384–93.

33. Ono K, Iijima T. Pathophysiological significance of T-
type Ca2+ channels: properties and functional roles
of T-type Ca2+ channels in cardiac pacemaking.
J Pharmacol Sci 2005;99(3):197–204.

34. DiFrancesco D, Tortora P. Direct activation of
cardiac pacemaker channels by intracellular cyclic
AMP. Nature 1991;351(6322):145–7.

35. Baruscotti M, Bucchi A, Difrancesco D. Physiology
and pharmacology of the cardiac pacemaker
("funny") current. Pharmacol Ther 2005;107(1):
59–79.

36. Borer JS, Fox K, Jaillon P, et al. Antianginal and anti-
ischemic effects of ivabradine, an I(f) inhibitor, in
stable angina: a randomized, double-blind, multi-
centered, placebo-controlled trial. Circulation 2003;
107(6):817–23.

37. Leoni AL, Marionneau C, Demolombe S, et al.
Chronic heart rate reduction remodels ion channel
transcripts in the mouse sinoatrial node but not in
the ventricle. Physiol Genomics 2005;24(1):4–12.

38. Barbuti A, Baruscotti M, DiFrancesco D. The pacemaker current: from basics to the clinics.
J Cardiovasc Electrophysiol 2007;18(3):342–7.

39. Shi W, Wymore R, Yu H, et al. Distribution and prevalence of hyperpolarization-activated cation channel (HCN) mRNA expression in cardiac tissues. Circ Res 1999;85(1):e1–6.

40. Schulze-Bahr E, Neu A, Friederich P, et al. Pacemaker channel dysfunction in a patient with sinus node disease. J Clin Invest 2003;111(10):1537–45.

41. Mangoni ME, Nargeot J. Genesis and regulation of the heart automaticity. Physiol Rev 2008;88(3):919–82.

42. Herrmann S, Stieber J, Stockl G, et al. HCN4 provides a 'depolarization reserve' and is not required for heart rate acceleration in mice. EMBO J 2007;26(21):4423–32.

43. Alig J, Marger L, Mesirca P, et al. Control of heart rate by cAMP sensitivity of HCN channels. Proc Natl Acad Sci U S A 2009;106(29):12189–94.

44. Dobrzynski H, Boyett MR, Anderson RH. New insights into pacemaker activity: promoting understanding of sick sinus syndrome. Circulation 2007; 115(14):1921–32.

45. Chandler NJ, Greener ID, Tellez JO, et al. Molecular architecture of the human sinus node: insights into the function of the cardiac pacemaker. Circulation 2009;119(12):1562–75.

46. Ju YK, Chu Y, Chaulet H, et al. Store-operated Ca2+ influx and expression of TRPC genes in mouse sinoatrial node. Circ Res 2007;100(11):1605–14.

47. Schram G, Pourrier M, Melnyk P, et al. Differential distribution of cardiac ion channel expression as a basis for regional specialization in electrical function. Circ Res 2002;90(9):939–50.

48. Joyner RW, van Capelle FJ. Propagation through electrically coupled cells. How a small SA node drives a large atrium. Biophys J 1986;50(6):1157–64.

49. Nof E, Luria D, Brass D, et al. Point mutation in the HCN4 cardiac ion channel pore affecting synthesis, trafficking, and functional expression is associated with familial asymptomatic sinus bradycardia. Circulation 2007;116(5):463–70.

50. Wang Q, Shen J, Li Z, et al. Cardiac sodium channel mutations in patients with long QT syndrome, an inherited cardiac arrhythmia. Hum Mol Genet 1995; 4(9):1603–7.

51. Vatta M, Dumaine R, Varghese G, et al. Genetic and biophysical basis of sudden unexplained nocturnal death syndrome (SUNDS), a disease allelic to Brugada syndrome. Hum Mol Genet 2002;11(3): 337–45.

52. Tan HL, Bink-Boelkens MT, Bezzina CR, et al. A sodium-channel mutation causes isolated cardiac conduction disease. Nature 2001;409(6823): 1043–7.

53. Schott JJ, Alshinawi C, Kyndt F, et al. Cardiac conduction defects associate with mutations in SCN5A. Nat Genet 1999;23(1):20–1.

54. Lei M, Huang CL, Zhang Y. Genetic Na+ channelopathies and sinus node dysfunction. Prog Biophys Mol Biol 2008;98(2-3):171–8.

55. Makita N, Sasaki K, Groenewegen WA, et al. Congenital atrial standstill associated with coinheritance of a novel SCN5A mutation and connexin 40 polymorphisms. Heart Rhythm 2005;2(10):1128–34.

56. Groenewegen WA, Firouzi M, Bezzina CR, et al. A cardiac sodium channel mutation cosegregates with a rare connexin40 genotype in familial atrial standstill. Circ Res 2003;92(1):14–22.

57. Cai J, Lin G, Jiang H, et al. Transplanted neonatal cardiomyocytes as a potential biological pacemaker in pigs with complete atrioventricular block. Transplantation 2006;81(7):1022–6.

58. Lin G, Cai J, Jiang H, et al. Biological pacemaker created by fetal cardiomyocyte transplantation. J Biomed Sci 2005;12(3):513–9.

59. Rosen MR, Robinson RB, Brink P, et al. Recreating the biological pacemaker. Anat Rec A Discov Mol Cell Evol Biol 2004;280(2):1046–52.

60. Xue T, Cho HC, Akar FG, et al. Functional integration of electrically active cardiac derivatives from genetically engineered human embryonic stem cells with quiescent recipient ventricular cardiomyocytes: insights into the development of cell-based pacemakers. Circulation 2005;111(1):11–20.

Progressive Conduction Diseases

Claire A. Martin, MB, BChir[a], Christopher L.-H. Huang, PhD[a], Andrew A. Grace, MB, PhD[b,c],*

KEYWORDS

- Conduction disease • Sodium channels • Arrhythmia
- Genetics

Conduction diseases encompass an important group of cardiac conditions that are potentially life threatening and account for approximately 50% of the 1 million permanent pacemakers implanted each year.[1] These diseases comprise a heterogeneous group of conditions that may be either inherited or acquired and may either be associated with structural abnormalities of the heart or manifest as primary electric diseases. The latter results from the presence of functionally abnormal or absent proteins, often cardiac ion channels involved in electric impulse generation.[2] This article reviews the causes of inherited functional cardiac conduction disease (CCD), particularly its more progressive forms.

The conduction system ensures rapid coordinated cardiac activation, which is initiated in the sinoatrial node, with the rate of depolarization dependent on the magnitude of the sodium current and thus on sodium channel function and availability. The depolarizing current then spreads between cells through intercellular gap junctions. These junctions each comprise hemichannels, each containing 6 connexin protein subunits.[3] Normal tissue function requires the molecular components involved in electrophysiologic activity, contractile function, and cell-cell adhesion to be positioned correctly within the cell and anchored to each other and to the cytoskeleton. Functional conduction disease can result from genetic defects in any of these proteins, as well

as in the ion channels themselves, and may additionally be associated with cardiomyopathy and other structural defects.

HISTORY

In 1761, Morgagni[4] first linked recurrent fainting episodes with a slow pulse in a family. Similar observations were later made by Adams[5] and Stokes.[6] The development of the electrocardiogram (ECG) at the end of the nineteenth century provided tighter definitions of related phenotypes by making electric recordings possible. The first known report of a syncopal attack combined with ECG recordings came from van den Heuvel,[7] who described a case of congenital heart block.

While several specific acquired causes of CCD had been recognized during the nineteenth century, such as diphtheria, rheumatic fever, congenital syphilis, and maternal connective tissue disease, the first recognition that CCD could be inherited was probably in 1901 by Morquio,[8] who described disturbance in cardiac conduction occurring in multiple members of the same family. Although most reports of congenital heart block have concerned affected siblings (and may have represented cases caused by circulating autoantibodies in the mother), the occurrence of the disease in 2 or more generations is often enough to prove inheritance.[9–11] Gazes and colleagues[12]

The British Heart Foundation, the Medical Research Council, the Wellcome, Trust, and the Biotechnology and Biological Research Council, UK provided funding. A Medical Research Council Clinical Research Fellowship and a Sackler Studentship of the University of Cambridge School of Clinical Medicine supported CAM.

a The Physiology Department, University of Cambridge, Downing Site, Cambridge CB2 3EG, UK
b Department of Biochemistry, University of Cambridge, Downing Site, CB2 1QW, UK
c Department of Cardiology, Papworth Hospital, Cambridge CB23 3RE, UK
* Corresponding author. Department of Biochemistry, University of Cambridge, Downing Site, CB2 1QW, UK.
E-mail address: ag@bioc.cam.ac.uk

reported conduction disturbances in 3 generations of a family.

EARLY DESCRIPTIONS OF PROGRESSIVE CCD

It was not until 1964 that 2 independent researchers published reports on a form of progressive CCD (PCCD) combining clinical observations, ECG recordings, and detailed postmortem studies of the heart.[13,14] Their descriptions were subtly different, with Lev[13] describing a diffuse fibrotic degeneration through the fibrous skeleton of the heart, whereas Lenegre[14] describing that the fibrosis was limited to the conduction fibers. However, both forms involved progressive conduction slowing through the His-Purkinje system with left bundle branch block (LBBB) or right bundle branch block (RBBB) and widening of QRS complexes, leading to complete atrioventricular (AV) block and sometimes causing syncope or sudden cardiac death (SCD). Lenègre-Lev syndrome is now synonymous with PCCD.

Although PCCD encompasses a heterogeneous group of conditions, the clear inherited component present in some families has led researchers to the causative genes. There have been several descriptions of CCD in families in South Africa. Combrink and colleagues[15] described a family in which the mother had RBBB and died suddenly and several other members displayed SCD and other conduction disturbances. In another family, 6 of 17 studied members showed a rhythm or conduction disturbance.[16] Brink and Torrington[17] referred to the disease as type I progressive familial heart block (PFHB). van der Merwe and colleagues[18,19] provided follow-up, demonstrating the progressive nature of the disease. A distinct clinical entity PFHB type II was also characterized, with complete heart block but narrow complexes. A similar disease was prevalent in Lebanon, with conduction defects, especially RBBB, which was progressive over time.[20,21]

THE ROLE OF SCN5A

The first gene to be associated with PCCD was SCN5A, which encodes the cardiac sodium channel Na$_v$1.5. Sodium channels are essential for the transmission of the cardiac impulse through both the fast conducting system and the working myocardium,[22] and therefore loss-of-function mutations would be expected to result in conduction disease. In 1999, Schott and colleagues[23] described a family with PCCD with various types of conduction disorders that displayed in its members RBBB, LBBB, left anterior or posterior hemiblock, and long PR intervals. These defects

were progressive over time (**Fig. 1**). Linkage analysis mapped the disease locus near SCN5A on chromosome 3. Direct sequencing of DNA of affected members identified a splice donor site mutation in exon 22 of SCN5A (IVS.22+2T->C) in 25 affected members. These observations suggest that PCCD associates SCN5A loss of function with an additional permissive factor related to aging.

Since then, there have been many reports identifying new SCN5A mutations causing PCCD or non-PCCD. Mutations have been found in various locations on SCN5A (**Fig. 2**) and have been postulated to cause loss of sodium channel function. In some, mutations result in a nonfunctioning protein,[24–26] whereas in others there is a defect in the trafficking mechanisms or in the channel gating behavior once the protein is inserted into the membrane.[27–32]

In the case of a Dutch family segregating a specific missense allele (G514C), the mutation causes unequal depolarizing shifts in the voltage dependence of activation and inactivation such that a smaller number of channels are activated at typical threshold voltages.[27] Two SCN5A mutations causing isolated conduction disturbances (G298S and D1595N) are also predicted to reduce channel availability by enhancing the tendency of channels to undergo slow inactivation in combination with a complex mix of gain- and loss-of-function defects.[29]

There are also cases in which individuals with severe impairment in conduction have inherited mutations from both parents. Lupoglazoff and colleagues[33] described a child homozygous for a missense SCN5A allele (V1777M) who exhibited rate-dependent AV conduction block. In a separate report, probands from 3 families exhibited perinatal sinus bradycardia progressing to atrial standstill (AS) (congenital sick sinus syndrome) and had compound heterozygosity for mutations in SCN5A.[34] Compound heterozygosity in SCN5A has also been observed in 2 cases of neonatal wide complex tachycardia and a generalized cardiac conduction defect.[28] These unusually severe examples of SCN5A-linked cardiac conduction disorders illustrate the clinical consequence of a near-complete loss of sodium channel function.

Recently, mutations having a modulator effect on SCN5A have been found. Niu and colleagues[35] described a W1421X mutation in a family in which 4 generations demonstrated cardiac conduction abnormalities and several cases of SCD. However, 1 member with the mutation was unaffected and was found to have a second mutation SCN5A-R1193Q postulated to have a protective

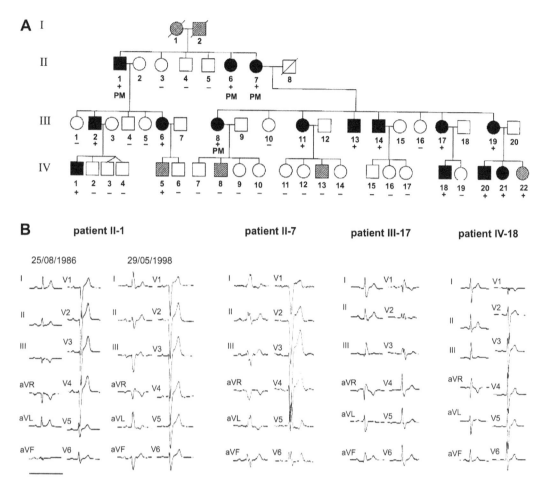

Fig. 1. (*A*) Pedigree of the French family identified by Schott and colleagues.[23] Patients with an unknown status (*stippled*) were not included in the linkage study. Individuals carrying the mutation are indicated with + as are patients with a pacemaker (PM). (*B*) Representative ECGs from the French family. Patient II-1 had an unspecified conduction defect (QRS duration 120 milliseconds) at the age of 60 years but left anterior hemiblock with wide QRS complexes and a long PR interval (240 milliseconds) at 72 years. ECGs from patients II-7, III-17, and IV-18 show complete LBBB, complete RBBB, and left posterior hemiblock, respectively. (*Adapted from* Schott JJ, Alshinawi C, Kyndt F, et al. Cardiac conduction defects associate with mutations in SCN5A. Nat Genet 1999;23:20–1; with permission.)

role in moderating the effect of the first mutation. Polymorphisms in connexin genes have also been found to have influence. Groenewegen and colleagues[36] identified *SCN5A-D1275N* cosegregating with 2 connexin 40 genotypes in familial AS. Whereas SCN5A-D1275N channels showed only a small depolarizing shift in activation compared with wild type, the combined effect led to the severe conduction defects.

All the above variants result in purely functional conduction disorders; however, *SCN5A* mutations may also result in structural abnormalities along with CCD. In 2004, a large family with members having sinus node dysfunction, arrhythmia, and ventricular dysfunction was found to harbor

SCN5A-D1275N,[37] demonstrating that genes encoding ion channels can also be associated with dilated structural phenotypes. Since then, other families with *SCN5A* mutations have been identified, who display heart failure and atrial arrhythmias as well as conduction disorder.[38–40] Although it is possible that such structural abnormalities arise through tachycardia-induced cardiomyopathy, most evidence suggests that dilated cardiomyopathy (DCM) may well be a primary manifestation of the *SCN5A* mutation.[41] This condition may result from interactions of the cardiac sodium channel with cytoskeletal components or through altered calcium homeostasis as a consequence of alterations in intracellular sodium concentrations.

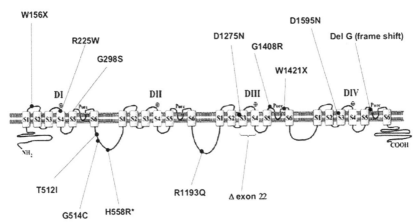

Fig. 2. Location of identified *SCN5A* mutations that result in conduction system disease. The asterisk indicates common polymorphism. (*Adapted from* Moric E, Herbert E, Trusz-Gluza M, et al. The implications of genetic mutations in the sodium channel gene (SCN5A). Europace 2003;5:325—34; with permission. For complete updated list of SCN5A variants associated with PCCD see http://www.fsm.it/cardmod/.)

Other sodium channel genes have also been implicated in CCD, such as *SCN1B*, which encodes the function-modifying sodium channel β1 subunit of the cardiac sodium channel.[42] Furthermore, a recent study has demonstrated cardiac expression of *SCN10A*, encoding the sodium channel Na$_v$1.8, and identified an association of a nonsynonymous single nucleotide polymorphism (SNP) in the *SCN10A* with prolonged cardiac conduction. The PR interval is shorter in *Scn10a*$^{-/-}$ mice than in wild-type mice, suggesting that SCN10A in humans acts to lengthen cardiac conduction and that this SNP in *SCN10A* is a gain-of-function variant.[43]

MOUSE MODEL OF PCCD

The authors' mouse model of Lenègre-Lev disease, an *Scn5a*$^{+/-}$ heterozygote, was generated through the replacement of exon 2 of the *Scn5a* gene with a splice acceptor (SA)-Gfp-PGK-neomycin cassette.[44] Whole cell patch clamp analyses of isolated ventricular myocytes from 8-to 10-week old heterozygous mice demonstrate that the cardiac sodium current is reduced by about 50% compared to wild-type mice (**Fig. 3**A, B).

The authors have shown in intact animal ECG recordings that the *Scn5a*$^{+/-}$ mice have several cardiac electric defects, including prolonged PR intervals, AV block, and prolonged QRS intervals (see **Fig. 3**C), that worsen with age (**Fig. 4**).[45] Monophasic action potential recordings[46] and activation mapping[47] have demonstrated delayed activation latencies, more pronounced in the right ventricle and worsening with age (see **Fig. 3**D, E). This age-dependent deterioration of ventricular conduction was associated with a pronounced

myocardial rearrangement, including fibrosis and redistribution of connexin 43 expression (**Fig. 5**). These observations demonstrate that a monogenic ion channel defect can lead, with aging, to myocardial structural anomalies. Thus PCCD may result from both a primary decrease in Na$^+$ current and a secondary progressive fibrosis and remodeling of connexin expression with aging. In this context, *Scn5a*$^{+/-}$ mice represent a potential tool for testing preventive therapies as an alternative or adjunctive approach to device implantation.

OVERLAP SYNDROMES

SCN5A mutations are associated not only with CCD but also with long QT 3 (LQT3) syndrome and Brugada syndrome (BrS). A gain-of-function mutation of the sodium channel is seen in LQT3 syndrome, leading to a long depolarizing current, prolonging the action potential.[48] BrS is associated with reduced Na$^+$ channel function and is characterized electrocardiographically by ST elevation in the right precordial leads and RBBB.[49]

Although isolated PCCD does not usually involve the ECG changes seen with BrS or LQT3 syndrome, *SCN5A* mutations may also be associated with more complex phenotypes that seem to represent combinations of the characteristics of BrS, conduction system disease, and LQT3 syndrome (**Fig. 6**). In 1 example, deletion of lysine-1500 in *SCN5A* was associated with not only impaired inactivation, resulting in a persistent Na$^+$ current, but also reduction in Na$_v$ channel availability by opposing shifts in voltage dependence of inactivation and activation.[50] These complex relationships between genotype and phenotype may underlie clinical findings that

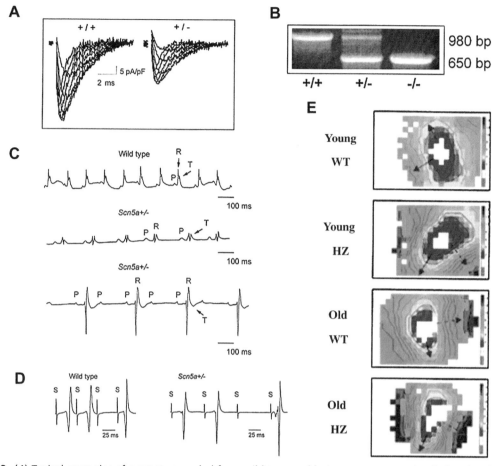

Fig. 3. (*A*) Typical examples of currents recorded from wild-type and heterozygous myocytes during depolarization steps from −100 mV to voltages between −50 and −15 mV in 5-mV increments. (*B*) PCR genotyping of E10.5 embryos identifying wild-type, *Scn5a*$^{+/-}$, and *Scn5a*$^{-/-}$ mice. (*C*) Representative single-lead ECG strips from wild-type (WT) and *Scn5a*$^{+/-}$ mice. For the WT mouse the cycle length is 120 milliseconds, with 1:1 conduction from atria to ventricles. The upper ECG taken from an *Scn5a*$^{+/-}$ mouse shows an increased cycle length of 220 milliseconds, with increased P-wave duration (26 milliseconds) and prolonged PR interval (60 milliseconds) when compared with WT. The lower ECG taken from an *Scn5a*$^{+/-}$ mouse shows second-degree atrioventricular block and prolonged PR interval (60 milliseconds) with a rightward shift in the QRS axis. (*D*) Characteristics of AV nodal conduction in WT and *Scn5a*$^{+/-}$ Langendorff-perfused hearts during right atrial pacing and left ventricular epicardial recording. Far-field atrial pacing stimulation artifacts (S) and resulting ventricular electrograms are shown. With the stimulus interval of the paced beats (S-S) progressively reduced for the WT heart, the third artifact that delivered at a stimulus interval of 42 milliseconds is not conducted to the ventricle. For the Scn5a1/_ mouse, AV conduction is significantly impaired, with the third atrial-paced beat (S) delivered at a stimulus interval (S-S) of 70 milliseconds not being conducted to the ventricle. (*E*) Representative activation maps of ventricles and atria. Depicted are the activation maps of the right ventricle of (*top panel*) young SCN5A WT, (*second panel from top*) young SCN5A heterozygous (HZ), (*third panel from top*) old SCN5A WT, and (*bottom panel*) old SCN5A HZ mice. Earliest activation is given in red, latest in blue. Black lines indicate the sites of isochronal activation; bold arrows, longitudinal conduction; dashed arrows, transversal conduction bp, base pair. (*Adapted from [A–D]* Papadatos GA, Wallerstein PM, Head CE, et al. Slowed conduction and ventricular tachycardia after targeted disruption of the cardiac sodium channel gene Scn5a. Proc Natl Acad Sci U S A 2002;99:6210–5; with permission; *[E]* van Veen TA, Stein M, Royer A, et al. Impaired impulse propagation in Scn5a-knockout mice: combined contribution of excitability, connexin expression, and tissue architecture in relation to aging. Circulation 2005;112(13):1927–35; with permission.)

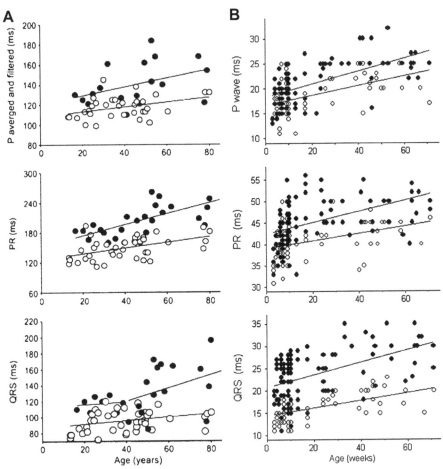

Fig. 4. (*A*) Evolution of conduction parameters in affected (*filled circles*) and unaffected subjects (*open circles*) with aging. (*Top panel*) averaged and filtered P-wave durations, (*middle panel*) PR duration, and (*bottom panel*) QRS duration. In the top and middle panels, data were fitted with a linear regression analysis. In the bottom panel, assessment of the residuals showed that the linear model was poorly adapted to fit the relation between QRS duration and aging in affected members. The variance was significantly different before and after the age of 40 years (ratio variance test; $P<.001$). This difference indicated a threshold effect of age. Thus, 2 linear regression analyses were performed before and after the age of 40 years. (*B*) Effects of age (x-axis) on P-wave duration (y-axis; *top*), PR-interval duration (y-axis; *middle*), and QRS-interval duration (y-axis; *bottom*) in wild-type (*open circles*; n = 106) and Scn5a$^{+/-}$ (*filled circles*; n = 85) mice. (*From* [A] Probst V, Kyndt F, Potet F, et al. Haploinsufficiency in combination with aging causes SCN5A-linked hereditary Lenègre disease. J Am Coll Cardiol 2002;41:643–52; with permission; [B] Royer A, van Veen TA, Le Bouter S, et al. Mouse model of SCN5A-linked hereditary Lenègre's disease: age-related conduction slowing and myocardial fibrosis. Circulation 2005;111(14):1738–46; with permission.)

individuals with BrS and an identifiable *SCN5A* mutation have longer PR intervals[51] and may experience more bradyarrhythmias[52] than individuals with BrS who do not have an identifiable *SCN5A* mutation. However, Lenègre-Lev syndrome and BrS remain 2 distinct clinical entities, because only those individuals with a BrS phenotype display ST elevation and ventricular arrhythmias.[53]

OTHER CANDIDATE GENES

Mutations in genes encoding other relevant proteins have been identified in families with conduction disorders, although these do not usually exhibit the progression with age seen in Lenègre-Lev syndrome. Furthermore, often mutations at the same site either may result in purely functional conduction defects or may also be

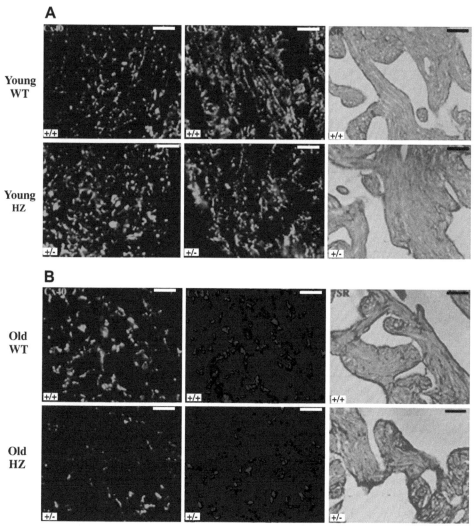

Fig. 5. Immunohistochemical staining of the atria in young (*A*) and old (*B*) mice. Left and middle panels show immunolabeling against Cx40 and Cx43, respectively (bar = 25 μm), whereas right panels show the presence of fibrosis (*red*) as marked with Sirius red (SR) staining (bar = 50 μm). Whereas Cx40 and Cx43 patterns in the young animals are comparable in wild-type (WT) and heterozygous (HZ) animals, both connexins are downregulated and redistributed in the old HZ animals. However, the amount of fibrosis in the old atria is similar in WT and HZ animals, even though it has increased with aging. +/+,WT; +/−, HZ. (*From* van Veen TA, Stein M, Royer A, et al. Impaired impulse propagation in Scn5a-knockout mice: combined contribution of excitability, connexin expression, and tissue architecture in relation to aging. Circulation 2005;112(13):1927–35; with permission.)

associated with DCM, restrictive cardiomyopathy, or other structural defects.

Several microsatellite markers in Lebanese families and type I conduction disorder seen in South Africa mentioned earlier have been mapped to chromosome 19q13.2–13.3[54,55] More recently, the genetic interval for the PFHB type I disease locus has been further refined, with a missense mutation in *TRPM4* isolated as the cause of blunted cardiac conduction in several branches of a large Afrikaner family.[56] *TRPM4* encodes a Ca^{2+}-activated channel in in vitro expression systems[57] and has been suggested to contribute to the transient inward current initiated by Ca^{2+} waves. The PFHB type I–associated mutation, which results in an amino acid sequence change in the TRPM4 N-terminus, was found to lead to constitutive sumoylation of TRPM4 and impaired TRPM4 endocytosis, resulting in a dominant gain of TRPM4 channel function (**Fig. 7**).

Mutations in *TBX5*, a T-box transcription factor, have been identified in patients with Holt-Oram syndrome, involving CCD and AF as well as cardiac septation defects and extracardiac abnormalities.[58]

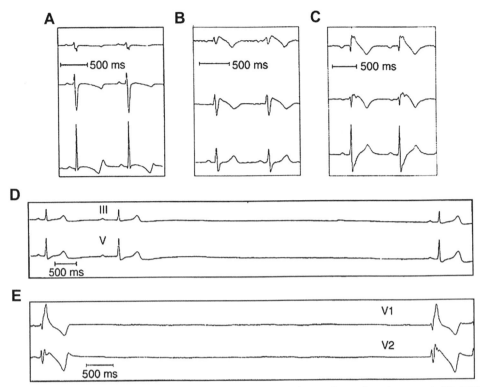

Fig. 6. ECG tracings of mutation carriers showing leads V_1, V_2, and V_5 unless otherwise stated. (A) QT-interval prolongation; (B) ST-segment elevation; (C) ST-segment elevation and RBBB; (D) First-degree AV block; (E) Sinus arrest. (*From* Grant AO, Carboni MP, Neplioueva V, et al. Long QT syndrome, Brugada syndrome, and conduction system disease are linked to a single sodium channel mutation. J Clin Invest 2002;110(8):1201–9; with permission.)

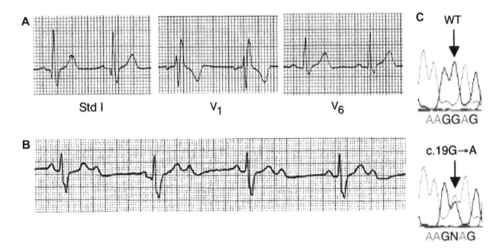

Fig. 7. Cardiac phenotype of patients with PFHB type I. (A) Sinus rhythm with RBBB in an 8-year-old asymptomatic boy on a standard 12-lead ECG, with leads Std I, V_1, and V_6 shown. (B) A 2:1 AV node block (atrial rate, 76 beats per minute; ventricular rate, 38 beats per minute) with a broad QRS complex on Holter monitoring in a 54-year-old man who had recently become symptomatic. ECGs were recorded at a 25-mm/s paper speed and 10-mm/mV signal amplitude. (C) TRPM4 missense mutation in exon 1 associated with PFHB type I. Electropherograms show TRPM4 wild-type (WT) sequence and the heterozygous sequence change c.19G→A in the DNA of PFHB type I–affected individuals. (*From* Kruse M, Schulze-Bahr E, Corfield V, et al. Impaired endocytosis of the ion channel TRPM4 is associated with human progressive familial heart block type I. J Clin Invest 2009;119(9):2737–44; with permission.)

NKX2.5 (cardiac-specific homeobox) mutations have also been identified in cases of CCD associated with septal defects[59] or tetralogy of Fallot.[60]

An intact cytoskeleton is required for proper myocyte structure and is involved in the cell signaling process. Mutations in genes encoding cytoskeletal proteins can lead to cardiomyopathy or muscular dystrophy, an example being the LMNA A/C gene, encoding laminin.[61] However, often the first and most prominent disease manifestation is isolated CCD, without or before the development of detectable structural cardiac abnormalities. It seems that mutations in cytoskeletal proteins directly or indirectly alter ion channel function. This finding is supported by recent studies showing that γ-syntrophin interacts with the α subunit of the cardiac sodium channel, thereby regulating its membrane expression and gating behavior.[62] Interactions of cytoskeletal proteins with mutant sodium channels may explain the exaggerated fibrosis seen in some cases of Lenègre-Lev syndrome.[26,28]

Mutations in *PRKAG2* encoding an AMP-activated protein kinase have been found in cases of both isolated CCD[63] and conduction disease with cardiac hypertrophy.[64] These mutations may influence cardiac conduction by affecting the phosphorylation state of several cardiac ion channels, such as T172D that is known to affect the inactivation properties of the human cardiac sodium channel in heterologous cell expression.[65]

Inborn errors of metabolism that affect normal transport and metabolism of fatty acids because of enzymatic defects may present as conduction disease and atrial arrhythmias without structural heart disease, although they can also be associated with cardiomyopathies. Usually, patients have defects in enzymes that regulate mitochondrial transport of long-chain fatty acids.[66] The accumulation of fatty acid metabolites downstream from the enzyme defect can be myotoxic and may also influence ion channels. These metabolites have been shown to reduce the inward rectifying K^+ and depolarizing Na^+ current, activate Ca^{2+} channels, and impair gap junction hemichannel interaction.[67]

SUMMARY

PCCD is a source of considerable morbidity and is likely to become more common with an aging population. This disorder represents a heterogeneous group of related conditions, mostly of unknown origin. It is likely that most cases are multifactorial. The progressive nature of the disease with age suggests that genetic environmental modifiers, and other imposed physiologic factors participate in disease expression.

Some cases point to monogenic inheritance, with the candidate *SCN5A* having been studied in most detail. Numerous mutations have been described, which are of variable penetrance and lead to a wide phenotypic spectrum. Whereas most mutations cause an isolated conduction disorder, some are associated with other arrhythmias and structural disease. A heterozygotic *Scn5a* mouse provides evidence that PCCD may involve cardiac remodeling along with conduction slowing. A range of other genes coding for proteins involved in impulse propagation have been implicated in progressive and nonprogressive conduction disorders, both in the presence or absence of structural abnormalities. Although currently pacemaker implantation is the usual treatment, once the pathophysiology of these diseases are more precisely identified other therapeutic approaches may be suggested.

REFERENCES

1. Adan V, Crown LA. Diagnosis and treatment of sick sinus syndrome. Am Fam Physician 2003;67(8): 1725.
2. Roden DM, Balser JR, George AL Jr, et al. Cardiac ion channels. Annu Rev Physiol 2002;64:431.
3. van Veen AA, van Rijen HV, Opthof T. Cardiac gap junction channels: modulation of expression and channel properties. Cardiovasc Res 2001;51(2):217.
4. Morgagni G. De sedibus, et causis morborum per anatomen indagatis libri quinque. 1761;2(1).
5. Adams R. Causes of disease of the heart, accompanied with pathological observation. Dublin Hosp Rep 1827;4:353.
6. Stokes W. Observations on some cases of permanently slow pulse. Q J Med Sci 1846;2:73.
7. van den Heuvel G. Die ziekte van stokes-adams en een geval van aangeborne hart blok. Groningen (The Netherlands) 1908.
8. Morquio L. Sur une maladie infantile et familiale caracterisee par des modifications permanentes du pouls, des attaques syncopales et epileptiformes et la mort subite. Arch Med Enfants 1901;4:467 [in French].
9. Wendkos M. Familial congenital complete A-V heart blocks. Am Heart J 1947;34:138.
10. Fulton Z, Judson C, Norris G. Congenital heart block occurring in a father and two children. Am J Med Sci 1910;140:339.
11. Wallgren A, Winblad S. Congenital heart-block. Am Heart J 1937;84:175.
12. Gazes PC, Culler RM, Taber E, et al. Congenital familial cardiac conduction defects. Circulation 1965;32:32.

13. Lev M. The pathology of complete atrioventricular block. Prog Cardiovasc Dis 1964;6:317.

14. Lenegre J. Etiology and pathology of bilateral bundle branch block in relation to complete heart block. Prog Cardiovasc Dis 1964;6:409.

15. Combrink JM, Davis WH, Snyman HW. Familial bundle branch block. Am Heart J 1962;64:397.

16. Steenkamp WF. Familial trifascicular block. Am Heart J 1972;84(6):758.

17. Brink AJ, Torrington M. Progressive familial heart block—two types. S Afr Med J 1977;52(2):53.

18. van der Merwe PL, Weymar HW, Torrington M, et al. Progressive familial heart block. Part II. Clinical and ECG confirmation of progression—report on 4 cases. S Afr Med J 1986;70(6):356.

19. van der Merwe PL, Weymar HW, Torrington M, et al. Progressive familial heart block (type I). A follow-up study after 10 years. S Afr Med J 1988;73(5):275.

20. Stephan E. Hereditary bundle branch system defect: survey of a family with four affected generations. Am Heart J 1978;95(1):89.

21. Stephan E, de Meeus A, Bouvagnet P. Hereditary bundle branch defect: right bundle branch blocks of different causes have different morphologic characteristics. Am Heart J 1997;133(2):249.

22. Herfst LJ, Rook MB, Jongsma HJ. Trafficking and functional expression of cardiac Na+ channels. J Mol Cell Cardiol 2004;36(2):185.

23. Schott JJ, Alshinawi C, Kyndt F, et al. Cardiac conduction defects associate with mutations in SCN5A. Nat Genet 1999;23(1):20.

24. Herfst LJ, Potet F, Bezzina CR, et al. Na+ channel mutation leading to loss of function and non-progressive cardiac conduction defects. J Mol Cell Cardiol 2003;35(5):549.

25. Kyndt F, Probst V, Potet F, et al. Novel SCN5A mutation leading either to isolated cardiac conduction defect or Brugada syndrome in a large French family. Circulation 2001;104(25):3081.

26. Probst V, Kyndt F, Potet F, et al. Haploinsufficiency in combination with aging causes SCN5A-linked hereditary Lenegre disease. J Am Coll Cardiol 2003;41(4):643.

27. Tan HL, Bink-Boelkens MT, Bezzina CR, et al. A sodium-channel mutation causes isolated cardiac conduction disease. Nature 2001;409(6823):1043.

28. Bezzina CR, Rook MB, Groenewegen WA, et al. Compound heterozygosity for mutations (W156X and R225W) in SCN5A associated with severe cardiac conduction disturbances and degenerative changes in the conduction system. Circ Res 2003;92(2):159.

29. Wang DW, Viswanathan PC, Balser JR, et al. Clinical, genetic, and biophysical characterization of SCN5A mutations associated with atrioventricular conduction block. Circulation 2002;105(3):341.

30. Viswanathan PC, Benson DW, Balser JR. A common SCN5A polymorphism modulates the biophysical effects of an SCN5A mutation. J Clin Invest 2003; 111(3):341.

31. Valdivia CR, Ackerman MJ, Tester DJ, et al. A novel SCN5A arrhythmia mutation, M1766L, with expression defect rescued by mexiletine. Cardiovasc Res 2002;55(2):279.

32. Akai J, Makita N, Sakurada H, et al. A novel SCN5A mutation associated with idiopathic ventricular fibrillation without typical ECG findings of Brugada syndrome. FEBS Lett 2000;479(1–2):29.

33. Lupoglazoff JM, Cheav T, Baroudi G, et al. Homozygous SCN5A mutation in long-QT syndrome with functional two-to-one atrioventricular block. Circ Res 2001;89(2):E16.

34. Benson DW, Wang DW, Dyment M, et al. Congenital sick sinus syndrome caused by recessive mutations in the cardiac sodium channel gene (SCN5A). J Clin Invest 2003;112(7):1019.

35. Niu DM, Hwang B, Hwang HW, et al. A common SCN5A polymorphism attenuates a severe cardiac phenotype caused by a nonsense SCN5A mutation in a Chinese family with an inherited cardiac conduction defect. J Med Genet 2006;43(10):817.

36. Groenewegen WA, Firouzi M, Bezzina CR, et al. A cardiac sodium channel mutation cosegregates with a rare connexin40 genotype in familial atrial standstill. Circ Res 2003;92(1):14.

37. McNair WP, Ku L, Taylor MR, et al. SCN5A mutation associated with dilated cardiomyopathy, conduction disorder, and arrhythmia. Circulation 2004;110(15): 2163.

38. Olson TM, Michels VV, Ballew JD, et al. Sodium channel mutations and susceptibility to heart failure and atrial fibrillation. JAMA 2005;293(4):447.

39. Laitinen-Forsblom PJ, Makynen P, Makynen H, et al. SCN5A mutation associated with cardiac conduction defect and atrial arrhythmias. J Cardiovasc Electrophysiol 2006;17(5):480.

40. Ge J, Sun A, Paajanen V, et al. Molecular and clinical characterization of a novel SCN5A mutation associated with atrioventricular block and dilated cardiomyopathy. Circ Arrhythm Electrophysiol 2008;1(2):83.

41. Bezzina CR, Remme CA. Dilated cardiomyopathy due to sodium channel dysfunction: what is the connection? Circ Arrhythm Electrophysiol 2008;1(2):80.

42. Watanabe H, Koopmann TT, Le Scouarnec S, et al. Sodium channel beta1 subunit mutations associated with Brugada syndrome and cardiac conduction disease in humans. J Clin Invest 2008;118(6): 2260.

43. Chambers JC, Zhao J, Terracciano CM, et al. Genetic variation in SCN10A influences cardiac conduction. Nat Genet 2010;42(2):149–52.

44. Papadatos GA, Wallerstein PM, Head CE, et al. Slowed conduction and ventricular tachycardia after targeted disruption of the cardiac sodium channel

gene Scn5a. Proc Natl Acad Sci U S A 2002;99(9): 6210.

45. Royer A, van Veen TA, Le Bouter S, et al. Mouse model of SCN5A-linked hereditary Lenègre's disease: age-related conduction slowing and myocardial fibrosis. Circulation 2005;111(14):1738.

46. Martin CA, Zhang Y, Grace AA, et al. Increased right ventricular repolarization gradients promote arrhythmogenesis in a murine model of Brugada syndrome. J Cardiovasc Electrophysiol 2010;21(10):1153.

47. van Veen TA, Stein M, Royer A, et al. Impaired impulse propagation in Scn5a-knockout mice: combined contribution of excitability, connexin expression, and tissue architecture in relation to aging. Circulation 2005;112(13):1927.

48. Stokoe KS, Thomas G, Goddard CA, et al. Effects of flecainide and quinidine on arrhythmogenic properties of Scn5a+/Delta murine hearts modelling long QT syndrome 3. J Physiol 2007; 578(Pt 1):69.

49. Brugada P, Brugada J. Right bundle branch block, persistent ST segment elevation and sudden cardiac death: a distinct clinical and electrocardiographic syndrome. A multicenter report. J Am Coll Cardiol 1992;20(6):1391.

50. Grant AO, Carboni MP, Neplioueva V, et al. Long QT syndrome, Brugada syndrome, and conduction system disease are linked to a single sodium channel mutation. J Clin Invest 2002;110(8):1201.

51. Smits JP, Eckardt L, Probst V, et al. Genotype-phenotype relationship in Brugada syndrome: electrocardiographic features differentiate SCN5A-related patients from non-SCN5A-related patients. J Am Coll Cardiol 2002;40(2):350.

52. Makiyama T, Akao M, Tsuji K, et al. High risk for bradyarrhythmic complications in patients with Brugada syndrome caused by SCN5A gene mutations. J Am Coll Cardiol 2005;46(11):2100.

53. Probst V, Allouis M, Sacher F, et al. Progressive cardiac conduction defect is the prevailing phenotype in carriers of a Brugada syndrome SCN5A mutation. J Cardiovasc Electrophysiol 2006;17(3):270.

54. Brink PA, Ferreira A, Moolman JC, et al. Gene for progressive familial heart block type I maps to chromosome 19q13. Circulation 1995;91(6):1633.

55. de Meeus A, Stephan E, Debrus S, et al. An isolated cardiac conduction disease maps to chromosome 19q. Circ Res 1995;77(4):735.

56. Kruse M, Schulze-Bahr E, Corfield V, et al. Impaired endocytosis of the ion channel TRPM4 is associated with human progressive familial heart block type I. J Clin Invest 2009;119(9):2737.

57. Launay P, Fleig A, Perraud AL, et al. TRPM4 is a Ca2+ activated nonselective cation channel mediating cell membrane depolarization. Cell 2002;109(3):397.

58. Vaughan CJ, Basson CT. Molecular determinants of atrial and ventricular septal defects and patent ductus arteriosus. Am J Med Genet 2000;97(4):304.

59. Schott JJ, Benson DW, Basson CT, et al. Congenital heart disease caused by mutations in the transcription factor NKX2-5. Science 1998;281(5373):108.

60. McElhinney DB, Geiger E, Blinder J, et al. NKX2.5 mutations in patients with congenital heart disease. J Am Coll Cardiol 2003;42(9):1650.

61. Kanada M, Demirtas M, Guzel R, et al. Cardiomyopathy and atrioventricular block in Emery-Dreifuss muscular dystrophy—a case report. Angiology 2002;53(1):109.

62. Ou Y, Strege P, Miller SM, et al. Syntrophin gamma 2 regulates SCN5A gating by a PDZ domain-mediated interaction. J Biol Chem 2003;278(3):1915.

63. Gollob MH, Seger JJ, Gollob TN, et al. Novel PRKAG2 mutation responsible for the genetic syndrome of ventricular preexcitation and conduction system disease with childhood onset and absence of cardiac hypertrophy. Circulation 2001;104(25):3030.

64. Gollob MH, Green MS, Tang AS, et al. Identification of a gene responsible for familial Wolff-Parkinson-White syndrome. N Engl J Med 2001;344(24):1823.

65. Light PE, Wallace CH, Dyck JR. Constitutively active adenosine monophosphate-activated protein kinase regulates voltage-gated sodium channels in ventricular myocytes. Circulation 2003;107(15):1962.

66. Saudubray JM, Martin D, de Lonlay P, et al. Recognition and management of fatty acid oxidation defects: a series of 107 patients. J Inherit Metab Dis 1999;22(4):488.

67. Bonnet D, Martin D, Pascale De L, et al. Arrhythmias and conduction defects as presenting symptoms of fatty acid oxidation disorders in children. Circulation 1999;100(22):2248.

Catecholaminergic Polymorphic Ventricular Tachycardia

Nicola Monteforte, MD[a], Marina Cerrone, MD[b],*

KEYWORDS

- Sudden cardiac death • Genetics • Ryanodine receptor
- CPVT • Calcium regulation

Catecholaminergic polymorphic ventricular tachycardia (CPVT) is one of the most malignant inherited arrhythmogenic diseases, with a high incidence of sudden cardiac death among affected individuals. The first report of a patient with this disease was published in 1975,[1] but the first systematic description came in 1978 with the work of Coumel and colleagues[2] and was further refined by the same group in 1995.[3] In 2001, molecular genetic studies[4–6] revealed that CPVT results from inherited defects of intracellular calcium handling proteins that cause abnormal Ca^{2+} release from the sarcoplasmic reticulum (SR). Our group reported for the first time that the autosomal dominant form of the disease was caused by mutations in the gene encoding for the cardiac ryanodine receptor.[4] Shortly after, the gene for the autosomal recessive form of CPVT was identified as the gene encoding cardiac calsequestrin.[5,6] After the identification of the underlying genetic causes, basic science studies in cell systems and animal models brought a major advancement to the understanding of arrhythmogenic mechanisms in this disease.

In the last few years, CPVT has attracted the interest of several investigators and the disease is now a well-characterized clinical entity.

In this article, the authors review the clinical and genetic aspects of CPVT and the main implications of mechanistic studies in the development of future therapeutic options for affected individuals.

GENETIC BASES

The genetic substrate of the 2 main forms of CPVT was discovered between 1999 and 2001 by linkage analysis and candidate gene screening. In 1999, Swan and colleagues[7] found a correlation with the chromosomal locus 1q42-q43 in 2 large families with CPVT. Subsequently, the authors' group discovered that the autosomal dominant form of CPVT is caused by mutations on the hRyR2 gene that encodes for the cardiac ryanodine receptor (RyR2).[4] The RyR2 is one of the proteins involved in the regulation of cardiac Ca^{2+} homeostasis. It controls the release of Ca^{2+} from the SR to the cytosol in response to the Ca^{2+} entry during the plateau phase of the action potential, as part of the Ca^{2+} induced-Ca^{2+} release process. Mutations in the RyR2 account, so far, for 55% to 60% of clinically diagnosed patients.

In 2001, Lahat and colleagues[5,6] reported a large Bedouin family affected by a recessive form of CPVT and harboring a mutation on the CASQ2 gene, encoding for calsequestrin. Calsequestrin is a buffering Ca^{2+} protein localized in the terminal cisternae of the SR; it participates together with triadin and junctin in modulating the responsiveness

There are no conflicts of interest to declare.
a Molecular Cardiology Laboratories, Fondazione S. Maugeri IRCCS, via Maugeri 10/10A, Pavia 27100, Italy
b Cardiovascular Genetics Program, Leon H. Charney Division of Cardiology, New York University School of Medicine, 522 First Avenue SRB707, New York, NY 10016, USA
* Corresponding author.
E-mail address: Marina.Cerrone@nyumc.org

cardiacEP.theclinics.com

of the RyR2 to luminal Ca^{2+} and controls the free Ca^{2+} concentration in the SR. At present, *CASQ2* mutations account for 3% to 5% of all genotyped patients. Aside from causing autosomal recessive CPVT, it is unclear whether *CASQ2* mutations may also cause an autosomal dominant transmission of the phenotype and cases of double heterozygosis in nonconsanguineous families have been reported.[8]

Recently, 2 other genes have been associated with a clinical spectrum consistent with CPVT.

Mutations on the *KCNJ2* gene have been described in individuals who had exercise-induced bidirectional ventricular tachycardia (VT) in the presence of normal QTc interval and without the extracardiac phenotype typical of patients affected by Andersen-Tawil syndrome, also caused by mutations on the same gene.[9] Additionally, preliminary in vitro data showed that the cellular mechanism of arrhythmias in *KCNJ2* mutants is similar to that described for *RyR2* and *CASQ2* mutants (see later discussion).[10]

Ankyrin B mutations have been recently described in few anecdotal cases showing clinical manifestations suggestive for CPVT, but further data are needed before considering systematic genetic screening in all patients with a suspect of CPVT.

ARRHYTHMOGENIC MECHANISMS: INSIGHTS FROM ANIMAL MODELS AND CELLULAR SYSTEMS

The effects of RyR2 and CASQ2 mutations have been studied in vitro and in vivo using different experimental models (expression in lipid bilayers, heterologous cell expression, and genetically engineered mouse models). The initial observation that bidirectional VT was observed in CPVT but also in cases of digitalis intoxication led investigators to propose that arrhythmias in CPVT could be caused by delayed after-depolarizations (DADs)-induced triggered activity. As a matter of fact, in the presence of digitalis toxicity, arrhythmias are elicited by DADs generated by the underlying intracellular Ca^{2+} overload.

There is general agreement that DADs-induced triggered activity caused by excessive diastolic Ca^{2+} release is the final substrate of arrhythmias in both forms of CPVT. However, multiple molecular mechanisms[11–13] have been invoked to explain how RyR2 mutations may disrupt cardiac Ca^{2+} homeostasis leading to intracellular Ca^{2+} overload and no univocal demonstration has been achieved. It is likely that different mutations may have different effects (mutation specific), ultimately resulting in the arrhythmic phenotype.

Genetically engineered mouse models have been useful to the understanding of the arrhythmogenic mechanisms of CPVT. The authors' group produced the first knock-in mouse model of CPVT, harboring the R4496C missense mutation that is associated with severe phenotype in patients.[14] Upon adrenergic stimulation this mouse model developed bidirectional and polymorphic VT whose morphology was close to the human arrhythmias. This finding led us to investigate the mechanisms of CPVT arrhythmias in this model. Initially, our group demonstrated that isolated ventricular myocytes from the $RyR2^{R4496C/WT}$ mouse show DADs and triggered activity if superfused with isoproterenol; whereas, wild-type cells do not.[15] Additionally, isolated $RyR2^{R4496C/WT}$ mouse Purkinje cells showed high inducibility of DADs and triggered activity, even in the absence of adrenergic stimulation.[16]

In isolated, Langendorff-perfused $RyR2^{R4496C/WT}$ mouse hearts, optical mapping experiments with a voltage-sensitive dye suggested that the arrhythmias in this model could originate from the specialized conduction system.[16] Optical maps during bidirectional VT showed the presence of alternating foci originating respectively from the left and the right ventricle, close to the epicardial site of emergence of the right and left bundle branch (**Fig. 1**). During polymorphic VT, optical maps of the right endocardial wall showed that the site of origin of different ectopic beats coincided with free-running Purkinje fibers.[16] The increased impairment in intracellular Ca^{2+} handling in mutant Purkinje cells derived from this model, if compared with ventricular myocytes, has been also supported by a recent series of experiments.[17,18] Isolated $RyR2^{R4496C/WT}$ Purkinje cells showed a higher tendency to develop spontaneous and larger Ca^{2+} release events if compared with ventricular myocytes; adrenergic stimulation increased the susceptibility of Purkinje cells to develop spontaneous Ca^{2+} waves, alternans, and sustained triggered activity, thus supporting the role of the specialized conduction system in initiating arrhythmias in this model.[17,18]

Several other mouse models harboring different RyR2 mutations have been generated and all supported the initial observation that arrhythmias are associated with DADs-induced triggered activity.[19,20]

Few *CASQ2* mutations have been reported so far. Most of them cause a premature truncation of the protein leading to haploinsufficiency. Few other missense mutations have been described; studies in cellular systems showed that they may cause the CPVT phenotype either by impairing the Ca^{2+} binding capacity of the protein or interfering with the inhibition of the RyR2.[8,20–22]

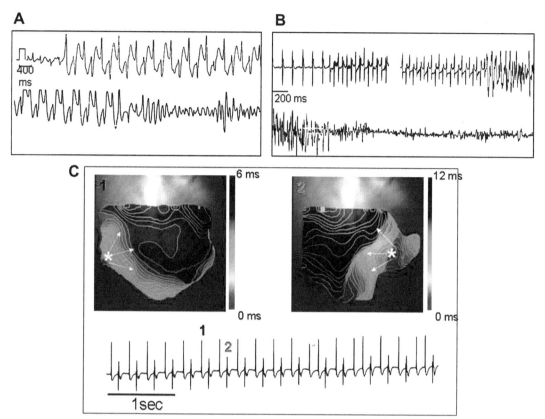

Fig. 1. (*A*) Bidirectional VT degenerating into ventricular fibrillation (VF) recorded in 1 patient affected by CPVT and carrier of the RyR2$^{R4497C/WT}$ mutation. (*B*) Bidirectional VT degenerating into polymorphic VT and ultimately into VF elicited by injection of caffeine and epinephrine in a RyR2$^{R4496C/WT}$ mouse. (*C*) Optical maps and volume-conducted ECG of bidirectional VT elicited in a Langendorff-perfused RyR2$^{R4496C/WT}$ mouse heart treated with isoproterenol. Map 1 and Map 2 correspond to beat 1 and beat 2, respectively.

Mouse models harboring homozygous *CASQ2* mutations are also available and they confirmed a common arrhythmogenic substrate for both forms of the disease.[23–25] However, these models also suggested interesting information about ultrastructural remodeling not previously observed in the RyR2 mutant mice. Knollman and colleagues[23] demonstrated a dramatic reduction in calsequestrin, triadin, and junctin levels in a CASQ2 knockout mouse model, associated with a compensatory increase in the volume of the SR, therefore avoiding a decrease in the SR Ca^{2+} content.

Similar ultrastructural abnormalities and a reduction in the calsequestrin levels were observed by the authors' group in a CASQ2$^{R33Q/R33Q}$ mouse model.[25] In this specific model, the mutation was provoking higher calsequestrin degradation by increased susceptibility to trypsin digestion.

Therefore, it becomes possible to speculate that, in analogy with what is hypothesized in RyR2-CPVT, different CASQ2 mutations may induce different functional abnormalities that lead to the common CPVT phenotype.

CLINICAL PRESENTATION AND NATURAL HISTORY OF CPVT

Patients with CPVT typically present with stress-induced syncope or sudden cardiac death.[3,4,26] Symptoms can occur in early childhood and the mean age of onset of the first syncope in the authors' large cohort of CPVT, recently confirmed in additional series, is 12 years.[26–28] In the absence of treatment, the disease is highly lethal, with an estimated incidence of sudden death before 40 years of age of 30%.[27] Growing evidence shows that sudden death may be the first manifestation of the disease, thus making prevention of lethal events a difficult task.

Frequently, patients with CPVT seek medical attention for the evaluation of unexplained syncope; in this setting, often they are misdiagnosed as being affected by vasovagal syncope or epilepsy because resting electrocardiogram (ECG) is normal. Minor, nondiagnostic features at rest are sinus bradycardia and prominent U waves (**Fig. 2**). Some investigators reported sinus bradycardia in some subjects with CPVT,[3,29] and Postma and colleagues[29] hypothesized that bradycardia may result from impaired Ca^{2+} handling by the mutant RyR2 channel in sinoatrial nodal cells. The presence of prominent U waves has also been reported,[30] but its diagnostic value has never been systematically evaluated and demonstrated. Furthermore, no significant abnormalities are identified at signal averaging electrocardiography and atrioventricular conduction is within normal limits, but a mild QT prolongation in some CPVT cases was reported.[3] Thus, CPVT

differential diagnosis should include long QT syndrome (LQTS). Patients with LQTS with a mild phenotype (borderline QT interval and no symptoms) do exist, but their prognosis is milder than that of CPVT, which presents a higher incidence of sudden death and a limited response to beta-blocker therapy.[26,31]

In the authors' series of subjects with CPVT, the presence of a positive family history for sudden death, stress-induced syncope, or seizures were present in 30% of subjects,[26] suggesting that careful collection of family history has an important role in leading toward the correct identification of this condition.

Independently from the clinical presentation (syncope or aborted sudden death), the most

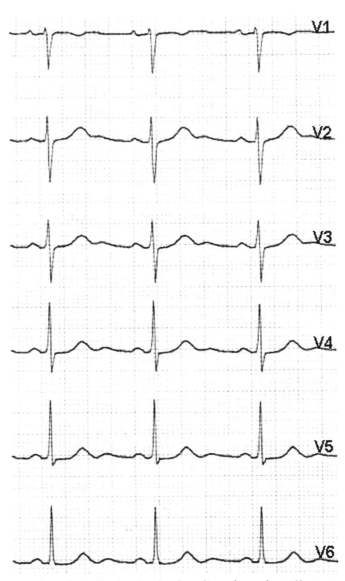

Fig. 2. Resting ECG in a patient with CPVT showing bradycardia and prominent U wave.

important clinical test to diagnose CPVT is the exercise stress test. In clinically overt CPVT (penetrant cases), there is a highly reproducible pattern of arrhythmias evoked during exercise stress test or isoproterenol infusion.[26,32] These observations enforce the concept that an exercise stress test should be performed in the routine evaluation of unexplained syncope, especially if adrenergic trigger is evident.

In a subset of patients, acute emotion represents a more powerful trigger than exercise. Hence, ECG-Holter monitoring and implantable loop recorders may be helpful for diagnosis in patients in whom emotional triggers (alone or in combination with exercise) are more arrhythmogenic than exercise alone.

The typical behavior of CPVT arrhythmias is that of a progressive worsening upon increase in workload; isolated premature beats or couplets initially appear at a critical rate of 90 and 110 bpm followed by runs of nonsustained or sustained VT when the heart rate further increases (**Fig. 3**). Supraventricular tachyarrhythmias are also part of the CPVT phenotype (see **Fig. 3**); one could speculate that fast supraventricular tachycardia may act as a trigger for development of DADs and triggered activity in the ventricle.[33] The morphology of VT is often the hallmark of the disease: the so-called bidirectional VT,[2,3,26] which is characterized by a 180°

beat-to-beat rotation of the axis of the QRS complexes on the frontal plane (**Fig. 4**). CPVT onset is mostly of single or double origin and usually originates from the right ventricular outflow tract; whereas, the ensuing beat tends to originate from the left ventricle.[33,34] Although this pattern is recognizable in the majority of patients, it is important to be aware that some patients also present irregular polymorphic VT. Furthermore, the initial presentation of the disease may also be adrenergically induced ventricular fibrillation (VF)[26] leading to the diagnosis of idiopathic VF. Since the early characterization of the disease, it has been evident that RyR2 mutations were present in a similar proportion among patients whose clinical presentation was bidirectional VT, polymorphic VT, or adrenergically induced idiopathic VF.[26,27] In genotype-phenotype correlations, it seems evident that the position of the specific mutation on the RyR2 does not correlate with the clinical presentation; therefore, individuals who carry the same mutation may present either bidirectional VT, polymorphic VT, or VF.[26]

Programmed electrical stimulation does not contribute to the clinical evaluation of patients with CPVT because ventricular arrhythmias are rarely inducible in CPVT. Conversely, epinephrine infusion may often induce the typical pattern of VT, although its diagnostic sensitivity does not

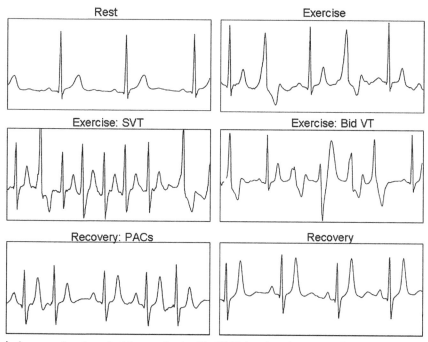

Fig. 3. ECG during exercise stress test in a patient with CPVT showing the onset of ventricular extrasystoles and their increase in frequency arrhythmias before the onset of supraventricular tachycardia and bidirectional VT. Bid VT, bidirectional VT; PACs, premature atrial complexes; SVT, supraventricular tachycardia.

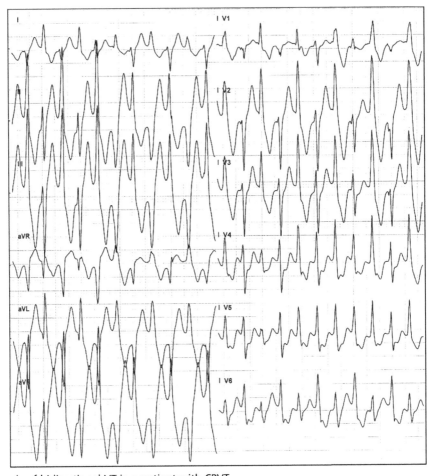

Fig. 4. Example of bidirectional VT in a patient with CPVT.

appear to be higher than that of an exercise stress test.

In 2002, the authors reported data showing that exercise/emotion-induced syncopal events occur in 67% of subjects; whereas, in 33% of families, juvenile sudden cardiac death was detectable.[26] These data were substantially confirmed by a Japanese group in 2003,[32] by another European study in 2005,[29] and by an analysis of our database on 119 subjects, which showed that close to 80% of these patients experience cardiac events before the age of 40 years.[27] This analysis demonstrated that in the absence of therapy, approximately 30% of these the patients have a first syncope or cardiac arrest before the age of 10 years; death or aborted cardiac arrest occur with an incidence close to 20% up to the age of 20 years.

Overall, these data highlight the severity of the disease and its almost complete penetrance demonstrated by a low percentage (20%) of asymptomatic carriers of mutations in the CPVT genes.[26,29] Therefore, on the basis of current

data, CPVT should be regarded as one of the most severe among inherited arrhythmogenic disorders.

Mutations in the RyR2 have been associated to an atypical form of Arrhythmogenic Right Ventricular Cardiomyopathy,[35] in which the arrhythmic phenotype seems to be more pronounced than the structural myocardial alterations. Additionally, in 2007, Bhuiyan and colleagues[36] described two unlinked families harboring a large deletion of the exon 3 of the RyR2. This family presented a wide spectrum of clinical symptoms aside from exercise-induced ventricular arrhythmias, including atrial bradyarrhythmias and tachyarrhythmias and mild, left ventricular dysfunction and dilatation. These reports led to the speculation that specific RyR2 mutations may not only disrupt Ca^{2+} homeostasis leading to increased propensity to arrhythmias but may also have an effect on the integrity of the myocardium; however, more detailed functional data are needed to understand which is the role played by RyR2 mutations in the setting of cardiomyopathies.

THE ROLE OF GENETIC TESTS IN THE CLINICAL MANAGEMENT OF CPVT

Genetic test in the setting of CPVT has a high positive yield and up to 70% of individuals with a clear phenotype are carriers of a mutation on the *RyR2* or *CASQ2* genes.[27] Early genetic evaluation is important for all family members of CPVT probands for presymptomatic diagnosis, identification of silent carriers, and appropriate reproductive counseling.

A positive genotype confirming the diagnosis of CPVT is essential in the clinical evaluation of patients and in the differential diagnosis.

So far, only a minority of patients have been found to carry mutations on the *KCNJ2* gene. Because this form appears to present a more benign course with lower incidence of sudden death, genetic screening on the gene *KCNJ2* appears reasonable in the absence of mutations on the two main genes.

Genetic test in CPVT is complicated by the fact that RyR2 is one of the largest genes in the human genome, with 105 exons, impacting turnaround time and accessibility.

As with other inherited arrhythmogenic diseases, CPVT involves a high degree of genetic heterogeneity with more than 70 mutations reported so far; most of them are private (ie, they are rare mutations present in a single family or in few probands). Therefore, mutation scanning of the open reading frame regions of *RYR2* and *CASQ2* is the most frequently used approach for mutation detection. Data from different groups showed that most of the CPVT-*RYR2* mutations cluster in specific regions of the protein: the N-terminal domain (amino acids 77-466), the FKBP12.6 binding domain (amino acids 2246-2534), and the transmembrane and C-terminal domains from amino acid 3778. Based on this observation, some laboratories have limited the screening on these selected regions, which includes, overall, 66 exons of the 105 total of the gene, and commercial companies have followed on these steps.[37] At variance with this approach, preliminary observations from the authors' large CPVT cohort (Priori SG, personal communication, 2010) show that 4% of *RYR2* probands have mutations outside of these clusters. Therefore, targeted exon analysis is likely to have lower detection sensitivity and carry implications in defining a partial test as negative. Considering that 20% of mutation carriers have no overt phenotype (incomplete penetrance) and sudden cardiac arrest can be the first clinical presentation in up to 62%[26,27] of cases, genetic screening for CPVT in cases of adrenergically mediated idiopathic VF is also advisable.

Until a few years ago, genetic tests were only performed by a few research laboratories. Recently, the availability of genetic screening through commercial companies has increased the accessibility of this tool to the medical community. These tests, however, carry significant costs and have raised the issue of reimbursement policies. The lack of rules and guidelines for the coverage of the costs of commercial genetic tests has limited the possibility of incorporating it into the clinical practice in several instances. In the attempt to address this issue, the authors' group has recently performed a cost-effectiveness analysis of genetic screening in inherited arrhythmias.[38] Performance analysis of genetic tests in the case of CPVT showed that the cost for one positive genetic test was $9170 and it was even reduced to $5263 for cases with a clear clinical diagnosis, in which the yield of genetic testing reached 62%. Therefore, in the presence of clear clinical phenotype, genetic test shows a good cost-effectiveness ratio for CPVT.

THERAPY

Based on the clear evidence of the critical role of adrenergic stimulation as a trigger for arrhythmias in CPVT, beta-blockers were proposed as the mainstay of CPVT therapy since the earlier reports on this disease[2,3] and they are indicated both for chronic treatment and for acute therapy of sustained ventricular tachycardia. Beta-blockers should be started immediately when CPVT is diagnosed. Agreement in the scientific community seems to indicate nadolol as the first choice among the available options for its once daily dosing and nonselective effect. Asymptomatic bradycardia should not be considered as a reason to reduce the dosage of beta-blocker therapy. The demonstration that triggered activity is induced by DADs and that DADs-induced arrhythmias are facilitated by faster heart rates provides a rationale to consider the heart rate slowing induced by beta-blockers as an additional antiarrhythmic action of the drug that acts in synergy with the inhibition of the sympathetic drive.[39]

In the published reports there is conflicting evidence on the long-term effectiveness of beta-blocking agents. Although Leenhardt and colleagues[3] and Postma and colleagues[29] have reported an almost complete prevention from recurrence of cardiac events with the exception of noncompliant patients, the authors[26] and others[28,32] observed recurrences of cardiac events or incomplete protection from exercise-induced arrhythmias in patients with CPVT treated with the maximally tolerated dose. In the Italian CPVT Registry, the incidence of recurrent arrhythmias while on therapy is as high as 30%.[26,27] In case of recurrences of syncopal episodes or sustained VT while on therapy, the implantable cardioverter-defibrillator (ICD) should be considered. The decision to implant an ICD needs to take into account the risks and potential complications associated with the young age of the patients[40]; moreover, the adrenergic surge that may follow the shock could trigger an arrhythmic storm leading to repeated discharges.[41] The management of patients with CPVT with an ICD requires careful programming of the device that considers the high incidence of supraventricular arrhythmias in these individuals as well as the potential deleterious effect of antitachycardic pacing in the setting of triggered arrhythmias. However, if medical therapy fails, the additional protection of the ICD, possibly implanted in a center with expertise in genetic arrhythmias, becomes pivotal in limiting the high lethality of this disorder. In the authors' series, up to 50% of subjects received an appropriate device intervention in a 2-year follow-up,[27] notwithstanding medical therapy. Of note, appropriate shocks were also recorded in subjects who were asymptomatic or showed syncope but not cardiac arrest before implanting the ICD.[27]

The incomplete protection afforded by beta blockers calls for the need of identifying new effective options. Calcium channel blockers, in particular verapamil, have been studied by Swan and colleagues[42] and Sumitomo and colleagues[32] in limited series of subjects. Rosso and colleagues[43] evaluated the efficacy of a combined association between beta blockers and verapamil. In this group, the combined treatment reduced or even suppressed the recurrences of exercise-induced arrhythmias or ICD shocks.

More recently, experimental data in a CASQ2 knock-out mouse model showed that flecainide, together with its Na^+ channel blocking effects, is able to directly block the RyR2.[44] In other CASQ2 mouse models, flecainide failed to show antiarrhythmic effects.[45] In the authors' RyR2$^{R4496C/WT}$ mouse model, flecainide was able to inhibit spontaneous Ca^{2+} release events especially in isolated Purkinje cells,[17] at a concentration lower than the one affecting the RyR2 channel open probability, suggesting that other mechanisms may interplay in preventing arrhythmias.

Watanabe and colleagues[44] reported suppression of arrhythmias in 2 subjects with CPVT when treated with oral flecainide. Even if data in larger series are needed before proposing the use of flecainide as medical treatment in CPVT, these results are worth further exploration.

Wilde and colleagues[46] provided preliminary evidence for long-term effectiveness of left sympathetic cardiac denervation (LCSD) in 3 subjects with CPVT and Scott and colleagues[47] reported a case of successful bilateral thoracoscopic sympathectomy. In the authors' experience, LCSD did not reach equally encouraging results and half of the subjects treated with this approach experienced, over a few years of follow-up, recurrence of stress-induced arrhythmias. Overall, LCSD does not guarantee full long-term antiarrhythmic protection and should not be considered an alternative to the ICD in case of failure of medical therapy; however, it is an important tool to limit and prevent arrhythmic storms or multiple ICD intervention in patients who are highly symptomatic.

Experimental Therapies for CPVT

Experiments in cell systems and CPVT animal models have been performed to explore new therapeutic possibilities. One strategy pursued by different groups was the identification of compounds able to act on the ancillary proteins participating in RyR2 regulation and thought to play a role in the arrhythmogenic effects of RyR2 mutations. Some RyR2 mutations are supposed to increase SR Ca^{2+} release by disrupting the interaction between the RyR2 and one of its regulatory proteins, called FKBP12.6. Therefore, some groups designed compounds (indicated as S107[18] or K201[19,44,48]) aimed specifically to restore the impaired interaction between the FKBP12.6 and the RyR2. Unfortunately, experimental data on the efficacy of these drugs in different animal models[15,19,48] yielded conflicting results, suggesting that more evidence is needed before suggesting their use in the clinical setting.

An alternative approach is to inhibit the effects of beta-adrenergic stimulation by acting on the downstream targets of RyR2 phosphorylation. CAMKII phosphorylates RyR2 at different sites during adrenergic activation. The pharmacologic inhibition of CAMKII is a promising approach. Moreover, it is known that CAMKII inhibition reduces both diastolic Ca^{2+} leakage and the transient inward current I_{ti} (the transmembrane current generating DADs). Preliminary observations from our in the RyR2$^{R4496C/WT}$ mouse model suggest that a specific CAMKII inhibitor, KN93,[49] could prevent arrhythmias both in vitro and in vivo, thus providing encouraging data toward novel therapeutic strategies involving this pathway.

SUMMARY

CPVT is a rare and lethal inherited form of arrhythmias that may cause sudden death caused by disruption of the cardiac Ca^{2+} homeostasis.

Such abnormal intracellular Ca^{2+} handling creates an unstable substrate that manifests primarily with the onset of arrhythmias upon adrenergic stimulation in the absence of macroscopic structural changes. Although uncommon, the in-depth analysis of CPVT pathophysiology is relevant to understand not only CPVT itself but also Ca^{2+}-mediated arrhythmogenesis in general. Considering that not all patients with a clinical diagnosis of CPVT carry mutations in RyR2 and CASQ2, it is clear that additional genes need to be identified and most likely their discovery will bring novel insights in the pathophysiology of the disease. Among the most pressing challenges for translational investigators is the development of novel therapeutic strategies to abate the burden of life-threatening events in affected children and young adults.

REFERENCES

1. Reid DS, Tynan M, Braidwood L, et al. Bidirectional tachycardia in a child. A study using His bundle electrography. Br Heart J 1975;37(3):339—44.
2. Coumel P, Fidelle J, Lucet V, et al. Catecholamine-induced severe ventricular arrhythmias with Adam-Stokes in children: report of four cases. Br Heart J 1978;40(Suppl):28—37.
3. Leenhardt A, Lucet V, Denjoy I, et al. Catecholaminergic polymorphic ventricular tachycardia in children. A 7-year follow-up of 21 patients. Circulation 1995;91(5):1512—9.
4. Priori SG, Napolitano C, Tiso N, et al. Mutations in the cardiac ryanodine receptor gene (hRyR2) underlie catecholaminergic polymorphic ventricular tachycardia. Circulation 2001;103(2):196—200.
5. Lahat H, Eldar M, Levy-Nissenbaum E, et al. Autosomal recessive catecholamine- or exercise-induced polymorphic ventricular tachycardia: clinical features and assignment of the disease gene to chromosome 1p13-21. Circulation 2001;103(23):2822—7.
6. Lahat H, Pras E, Olender T, et al. A missense mutation in a highly conserved region of CASQ2 is associated with autosomal recessive catecholamine-induced polymorphic ventricular tachycardia in Bedouin families from Israel. Am J Hum Genet 2001;69(6):1378—84.
7. Swan H, Piippo K, Viitasalo M, et al. Arrhythmic disorder mapped to chromosome 1q42-q43 causes malignant polymorphic ventricular tachycardia in structurally normal hearts. J Am Coll Cardiol 1999;34(7):2035—42.
8. di Barletta MR, Viatchenko-Karpinski S, Nori A, et al. Clinical phenotype and functional characterization of CASQ2 mutations associated with catecholaminergic polymorphic ventricular tachycardia. Circulation 2006;114(10):1012—9.
9. Tester DJ, Arya P, Will M, et al. Genotypic heterogeneity and phenotypic mimicry among unrelated patients referred for catecholaminergic polymorphic ventricular tachycardia genetic testing. Heart Rhythm 2006;3(7):800—5.
10. Ruan Y, Boveri L, Rossenbacker T, et al. Arrhythmogenesis in mutant KCNJ2 associated catecholaminergic polymorphic ventricular tachycardia. Circulation 2008;118:S525.
11. Jiang D, Xiao B, Yang D, et al. RyR2 mutations linked to ventricular tachycardia and sudden death reduce the threshold for store-overload-induced Ca2+ release (SOICR). Proc Natl Acad Sci U S A 2004;101(35):13062—7.
12. Oda T, Yano M, Yamamoto T, et al. Defective regulation of interdomain interactions within the ryanodine receptor plays a key role in the pathogenesis of heart failure. Circulation 2005;111(25):3400—10.
13. Wehrens XH, Lehnart SE, Huang F, et al. FKBP12.6 deficiency and defective calcium release channel (ryanodine receptor) function linked to exercise-induced sudden cardiac death. Cell 2003;113(7):829—40.
14. Cerrone M, Colombi B, Santoro M, et al. Bidirectional ventricular tachycardia and fibrillation elicited in a knock-in mouse model carrier of a mutation in the cardiac ryanodine receptor. Circ Res 2005;96(10):e77—82.
15. Liu N, Colombi B, Memmi M, et al. Arrhythmogenesis in catecholaminergic polymorphic ventricular tachycardia: insights from a RyR2 R4496C knock-in mouse model. Circ Res 2006;99(3):292—8.
16. Cerrone M, Noujaim SF, Tolkacheva EG, et al. Arrhythmogenic mechanisms in a mouse model of catecholaminergic polymorphic ventricular tachycardia. Circ Res 2007;101(10):1039—48.
17. Kang G, Giovannone SF, Liu N, et al. Purkinje cells from ryr2 mutant mice are highly arrhythmogenic but responsive to targeted therapy. Circ Res 2010;107(4):512—9.
18. Herron TJ, Milstein ML, Anumonwo J, et al. Purkinje cell calcium dysregulation is the cellular mechanism that underlies catecholaminergic polymorphic ventricular tachycardia. Heart Rhythm 2010;7(8):1122—8.
19. Lehnart SE, Mongillo M, Bellinger A, et al. Leaky Ca2+ release channel/ryanodine receptor 2 causes seizures and sudden cardiac death in mice. J Clin Invest 2008;118(6):2230—45.
20. Kannankeril PJ, Mitchell BM, Goonasekera SA, et al. Mice with the R176Q cardiac ryanodine receptor mutation exhibit catecholamine-induced ventricular tachycardia and cardiomyopathy. Proc Natl Acad Sci U S A 2006;103(32):12179—84.
21. Terentyev D, Nori A, Santoro M, et al. Abnormal interactions of calsequestrin with the ryanodine receptor calcium release channel complex linked to exercise-induced sudden cardiac death. Circ Res 2006;98(9):1151—8.

22. Viatchenko-Karpinski S, Terentyev D, Gyorke I, et al. Abnormal calcium signaling and sudden cardiac death associated with mutation of calsequestrin. Circ Res 2004;94(4):471–7.

23. Knollmann BC, Chopra N, Hlaing T, et al. Casq2 deletion causes sarcoplasmic reticulum volume increase, premature Ca2+ release, and catecholaminergic polymorphic ventricular tachycardia. J Clin Invest 2006;116(9):2510–20.

24. Song L, Alcalai R, Arad M, et al. Calsequestrin 2 (CASQ2) mutations increase expression of calreticulin and ryanodine receptors, causing catecholaminergic polymorphic ventricular tachycardia. J Clin Invest 2007;117(7):1814–23.

25. Rizzi N, Liu N, Napolitano C, et al. Unexpected structural and functional consequences of the R33Q homozygous mutation in cardiac calsequestrin: a complex arrhythmogenic cascade in a knock in mouse model. Circ Res 2008;103(3):298–306.

26. Priori SG, Napolitano C, Memmi M, et al. Clinical and molecular characterization of patients with catecholaminergic polymorphic ventricular tachycardia. Circulation 2002;106(1):69–74.

27. Cerrone M, Colombi B, Bloise R, et al. Clinical and molecular characterization of a large cohort of patients affected with catecholaminergic polymorphic ventricular tachycardia. Circulation 2004;110 (Suppl):552.

28. Hayashi M, Denjoy I, Extramiana F, et al. Incidence and risk factors of arrhythmic events in catecholaminergic polymorphic ventricular tachycardia. Circulation 2009;119(18):2426–34.

29. Postma AV, Denjoy I, Kamblock J, et al. Catecholaminergic polymorphic ventricular tachycardia: RYR2 mutations, bradycardia, and follow up of the patients. J Med Genet 2005;42(11):863–70.

30. Aizawa Y, Komura S, Okada S, et al. Distinct U wave changes in patients with catecholaminergic polymorphic ventricular tachycardia (CPVT). Int Heart J 2006;47(3):381–9.

31. Priori SG, Napolitano C, Schwartz PJ, et al. Association of long QT syndrome loci and cardiac events among patients treated with beta-blockers. JAMA 2004;292(11):1341–4.

32. Sumitomo N, Harada K, Nagashima M, et al. Catecholaminergic polymorphic ventricular tachycardia: electrocardiographic characteristics and optimal therapeutic strategies to prevent sudden death. Heart 2003;89(1):66–70.

33. Monteforte N, Raytcheva-Buono E, Bloise R, et al. Electrocardiographic analysis of arrhythmias developing during exercise in patients with catecholaminergic polymorphic ventricular tachycardia. Circulation 2007;116(II):492.

34. Sumitomo N, Sakurada H, Taniguchi K, et al. Association of atrial arrhythmia and sinus node dysfunction in patients with catecholaminergic polymorphic ventricular tachycardia. Circ J 2007;71(10):1606–9.

35. Tiso N, Stephan DA, Nava A, et al. Identification of mutations in the cardiac ryanodine receptor gene in families affected with arrhythmogenic right ventricular cardiomyopathy type 2 (ARVD2). Hum Mol Genet 2001;10(3):189–94.

36. Bhuiyan ZA, van den Berg MP, van Tintelen JP, et al. Expanding spectrum of human RYR2-related disease: new electrocardiographic, structural, and genetic features. Circulation 2007;116(14):1569–76.

37. Medeiros-Domingo A, Bhuiyan ZA, Tester DJ, et al. The RYR2-encoded ryanodine receptor/calcium release channel in patients diagnosed previously with either catecholaminergic polymorphic ventricular tachycardia or genotype negative, exercise-induced long QT syndrome: a comprehensive open reading frame mutational analysis. J Am Coll Cardiol 2009;54(22):2065–74.

38. Rong B, Napolitano C, Bloise R, et al. Yield of genetic screening in inherited cardiac channelopathies: how to prioritize access to genetic testing. Circ Arrhythm Electrophysiol 2009;2:6–15.

39. Rosen MR, Danilo P Jr. Effects of tetrodotoxin, lidocaine, verapamil, and AHR-2666 on Ouabain-induced delayed after depolarizations in canine Purkinje fibers. Circ Res 1980;46(1):117–24.

40. Korte T, Koditz H, Niehaus M, et al. High incidence of appropriate and inappropriate ICD therapies in children and adolescents with implantable cardioverter defibrillator. Pacing Clin Electrophysiol 2004;27(7):924–32.

41. Mohamed U, Gollob MH, Gow RM, et al. Sudden cardiac death despite an implantable cardioverter-defibrillator in a young female with catecholaminergic ventricular tachycardia. Heart Rhythm 2006;3(12):1486–9.

42. Swan H, Laitinen P, Kontula K, et al. Calcium channel antagonism reduces exercise-induced ventricular arrhythmias in catecholaminergic polymorphic ventricular tachycardia patients with RyR2 mutations. J Cardiovasc Electrophysiol 2005;16(2):162–6.

43. Rosso R, Kalman JM, Rogowski O, et al. Calcium channel blockers and beta-blockers versus beta-blockers alone for preventing exercise-induced arrhythmias in catecholaminergic polymorphic ventricular tachycardia. Heart Rhythm 2007;4(9):1149–54.

44. Watanabe H, Chopra N, Laver D, et al. Flecainide prevents catecholaminergic polymorphic ventricular tachycardia in mice and humans. Nat Med 2009;15(4):380–3.

45. Katz G, Khoury A, Kurtzwald E, et al. Optimizing CPVT therapy in calsequestrin-mutant mice. Heart Rhythm 2010. [Epub ahead of print].

46. Wilde AA, Bhuiyan ZA, Crotti L, et al. Left cardiac sympathetic denervation for catecholaminergic polymorphic ventricular tachycardia. N Engl J Med 2008;358(19):2024–9.

47. Scott PA, Sandilands AJ, Morris GE, et al. Successful treatment of catecholaminergic polymorphic ventricular tachycardia with bilateral thoracoscopic sympathectomy. Heart Rhythm 2008;5(10):1461–3.

48. Wehrens XH, Lehnart SE, Reiken SR, et al. Protection from cardiac arrhythmia through ryanodine receptor-stabilizing protein calstabin2. Science 2004;304(5668):292–6.

49. Liu N, Colombi B, Napolitano C, et al. Ca^{2+}/calmodulin kinase II inhibitor abolishes and prevents triggered activity in myocytes from $RyR2^{R4496C+/-}$ knock-in mice. Heart Rhythm 2007;4(Suppl):S107–8.

Brugada Syndrome 2010

Paola Berne, MD*, Josep Brugada, MD, PhD

KEYWORDS

- Brugada syndrome • Channelopathies
- Inherited arrhythmias • Ventricular fibrillation
- Sudden cardiac death
- Implantable cardioverter-defibrillator

The syndrome of right bundle branch block (BBB), persistent ST-segment elevation, and sudden cardiac death (from polymorphic ventricular tachycardia [PVT] or ventricular fibrillation [VF]) in the absence of structural heart disease, which is currently known worldwide as *Brugada syndrome* (BS), was first described in 1992 by Pedro and Josep Brugada.[1] Since this first report, this rare, although potentially lethal disease affecting young and apparently healthy individuals, has attracted great interest from scientists and practitioners worldwide, resulting in a geometric increase of studies and scientific publications on the matter. This article briefly reviews recent advances in understanding of the syndrome's genetic and molecular basis, arrhythmogenic mechanisms, and clinical course, and an update of tools for risk stratification and treatment of the condition.

EPIDEMIOLOGY AND GENERAL CHARACTERISTICS

Some factors converge to make the estimation of BS prevalence difficult, including the variable penetrance of the disease, resulting in a high number of patients presenting concealed forms of the syndrome. Its presentation also has a marked geographic and ethnic variability. The estimated prevalence is believed to range from 1 to 5 cases/10,000 population in Europe[2–4] to 12 cases/10,000 population in Southeast Asia[5] (where it is considered endemic). When accounting for these factors, it appears that the real prevalence of BS is, in fact, higher.

The mean age at diagnosis in most series is 40 to 45 years (although BS has been identified in patients as young as 2 days old and as old as 84 years).[6] Most of the arrhythmic events also occur during the third and fourth decades of life,[7–12] and occur mainly during sleep or rest, or after large meals.

All published series clearly show a clear prevalence of men among affected individuals representing approximately 80% of patients.[7,8,10–12] The postulated theories regarding gender difference in BS are explained in further detail in the later discussion of cellular and ionic mechanisms underlying BS phenotype.

BS is thought to be responsible for 4% of all sudden deaths and up to 20% of sudden deaths in patients without cardiac structural disease.[6] It also has been recognized to be the same entity as sudden unexpected nocturnal death syndrome (SUNDS).[13] Evidence also links BS to sudden infant death syndrome (SIDS).[14,15]

GENETIC BASIS OF BRUGADA SYNDROME

BS is an inherited condition, transmitted in an autosomal-dominant way that presents variable penetrance. To date, mutations in eight genes have been linked to BS (**Table 1**).

The first identified causative gene was *SCN5A*,[16] which encodes for the pore-forming α-subunit of the cardiac sodium (Na^+) channel.

The authors have nothing to disclose.

Arrhythmia Section, Cardiology Department, Thorax Institute, Hospital Clínic, Institut de Investigació Biomèdica August Pi i Sunyer (IDIBAPS), University of Barcelona, C/Villarroel, 170, 08036 Barcelona, Catalonia, Spain
* Corresponding author.
E-mail address: pmberne@clinic.ub.es

Card Electrophysiol Clin 2 (2010) 533–549
doi:10.1016/j.ccep.2010.09.005

Table 1
Identified genes linked to Brugada syndrome

Gene	Chromosomal Location	Encoded Protein	Ionic Channel	Ionic Current	Functional Effect	Inheritance	% of Carriers Among BS Patients	Reference
SCN5A	3p21	Nav1.5	α-subunit I_{Na}	I_{Na}	Loss of function	Autosomal dominant	11–28	Chen et al[16]
GPD-1L	3p24	G3PD1L	Interaction with α-subunit I_{Na}	I_{Na}	Loss of function	Autosomal dominant	Unknown	London et al[18]
CACNA1C	12p13.3	Ca$_v$1.2	α-subunit I_{Ca}	I_{Ca}	Loss of function	Autosomal dominant	unknown	Antzelevitch et al[19]
CACNB2	10p12	Ca$_v\beta$2	β-subunit I_{Ca}	I_{Ca}	Loss of function	Autosomal dominant	Unknown	Antzelevitch et al[19]
SCN1B	19q13.1	Na$_v\beta$	β-subunit I_{Na}	I_{Na}	Loss of function	Autosomal dominant	Unknown	Watanabe H et al[21]
KCNE3	11q13.4	MiRP2	β-subunit I_{Ks}/I_{to}	I_{Ks}/I_{to}	Gain of function	Autosomal dominant	Unknown	Delpon et al[20]
SCN3B	11q23.3	Na$_v\beta$3	β-subunit I_{Na}	I_{Na}	Loss of function	Autosomal dominant	Unknown	Hu et al[22]
KCNJ8	12p11.23	K$_{ir}$6.1	K_{ATP} Kir6.1	IK_{ATP}	Gain of function	Autosomal dominant	Unknown	Medeiros-Domingo et al[23]

Mutations in *SCN5A* resulting in loss of function of the mentioned channel through different mechanisms are the most common genotype found among these patients (approximately 20% of BS case; range, 11%–28%). To date, almost 300 mutations in *SCN5A* have been described in association with BS.[17]

The second gene linked to BS[18] was glycerol-3-phosphate dehydrogenase 1-like gene (*GPD1L*). Mutations in *GPD1L*, leading to an abnormal trafficking of the cardiac Na^+ channel to the cell surface and causing a reduction of approximately 50% of the inward Na^+ current, also result in BS phenotype.

Mutations in genes encoding the $\alpha 1$ (*CACNA1C*) and β (*CACNB2b*) subunits of the L-type cardiac calcium (Ca^{+2}) channel, leading to a decrease of the ICa current, result in a combined Brugada/short QT syndrome. This finding was the first report of a mutation in a gene not affecting the cardiac Na^+ current being responsible for BS.[19]

More recently, mutations in KCNE3 gene (which encodes MiRP2, a protein that decreases the potassium (K^+) transient outward current (Ito) by interacting with channel Kv4.3), result in an increase of Ito magnitude and density, and produce BS.[20]

Mutations in SCN1B gene (encoding for $\beta 1$- and $\beta 1b$- subunits, auxiliary function-modifying subunits of the cardiac Na^+ channel, that normally increase the INa current), resulted in a decrease of the INa current by affecting the Na^+ channel trafficking.[21]

Mutations in SCN3B gene (which encodes for the $\beta 3$-subunit of the Na^+ cardiac channel) and leading to a loss-of-function of the Na^+ cardiac channel also cause BS.[22]

The last gene linked to BS is *KCNJ8*, which encodes the α-subunit of the cardiac ATP-sensitive potassium channel (K_{ATP} Kir6.1 channel, which has a preferential epicardial distribution). In a recent publication, Medeiros-Domingo and colleagues[23] found the missense mutation *S422L* resulting in a gain-of-function of the K_{ATP} Kir6.1 channel in 1 of 87 patients with BS, and also in 1 of 14 patients with early repolarization syndrome.

The percentage of BS patients carrying mutations in the last 7 causative genes has not been established yet. What seems clear is that the syndrome has a heterogeneous genetic basis, and that the number of genetic defects responsible likely will continue to increase.

Even if the percentage of patients who have a causative mutation is still low, and the availability and cost of genetic tests are prohibitive for most centers, the finding of a causative mutation in these genes undeniably implies diagnosis of the disease, and therefore identification of genetic mutations linked to BS should be included in the list of diagnostic criteria.

CORRECT RECOGNITION OF THE DIAGNOSTIC BRUGADA ELECTROCARDIOGRAM PATTERN

Three repolarization patterns have been associated with BS,[24] when found in the right precordial leads (ie, V_1 to V_3) (**Fig. 1**) and, less frequently, in the inferior leads (ie, DII, DIII and aVF).[25] Type I is characterized by a prominent coved ST-segment elevation displaying J point amplitude or ST-segment elevation of 2 mm or greater, followed by a negative T wave. Type II has a 2 mm or greater J point elevation, 1 mm or greater ST-segment elevation, and a saddleback appearance, followed

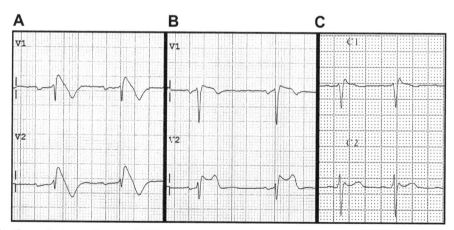

Fig. 1. The three electrocardiogram (ECG) patterns associated with BS. (*A*) Type I ECG. (*B*) Type II ECG. (*C*) Type III ECG.

by a positive or biphasic T-wave. Type III has either a saddleback or a coved appearance, but with an ST-segment elevation of less than 1 mm.

Even when the initial description included right RBBB as part of the required electrocardiogram (ECG) criteria, further studies established that right BBB may be associated with BS, but it is not an integral part of the disease.[26,27]

Type I is the only ECG diagnostic pattern of BS, whereas types II and III should be considered only suggestive of the disease.

According to the 2002 and 2005 consensus on BS, ECG diagnosis is reached when the pattern is found in at least two right precordial leads (V_1 to V_3); however, a recent study of 186 individuals diagnosed with BS found that V_3 did not yield diagnostic information in this group, and that patients showing a type I ECG in only one right precordial lead (V_1 or V_2) presented a similar clinical profile and arrhythmic risk to BS patients, with the same ECG pattern in more than one precordial lead.[28] These results may lead to a review of the current diagnostic criteria, requiring a type I ECG sign in only one right precordial lead for diagnosis.

DIAGNOSTIC TESTS IN BRUGADA SYNDROME

Several studies have informed about the dynamic character of the ECG in BS.[29,30] The three ECG patterns may coexist in the same patient (at different moments), and patients may even present normal ECGs that are only unmasked by fever, vagotonic agents, or class I antiarrhythmic drugs (AADs).[31] The ability of class I AADs to reproduce the diagnostic ECG pattern when administered to patients in whom the ECG

spontaneously normalized led to the use of these drugs as a diagnostic test in cases of suspected BS (**Fig. 2**). Drug challenge for diagnosis of BS is indicated when the disease is suspected but the basal ECG is normal (eg, familial screening) or suspicious, although not diagnostic (types 2 or 3). Flecainide, ajmaline, procainamide, disopyramide, propafenone, and pilsicainide have been used to unmask BS. **Table 2** outlines the current recommendations on drugs, doses, route, and time of administration. Drug challenge is only considered positive when a conversion to the diagnostic type I occurs.

Hong and colleagues[32] and Meregalli and colleagues[33] established the value of the two main pharmacologic tests used for diagnosing BS in patients with a causative *SCN5A* mutation. Ajmaline showed a sensitivity of 80%, specificity of 94%, positive predictive value of 93%, and negative predictive value of 83%, increasing the penetrance of the disease from 32.7 to 78.6%. Flecainide had a sensitivity of 77%, specificity of 80%, positive predictive value of 96%, and negative predictive value of 36%. The low negative predictive value of flecainide test, together with its short half-life makes ajmaline the preferred drug for diagnostic testing in cases of suspected BS, especially during family screening (**Fig. 3**).

During basal ECG and at the beginning and the end of the drug challenge test with class I AADs, placing the right precordial leads up to the third and second intercostal spaces is recommended because this increases the sensitivity of the ECG for detecting the diagnostic BS pattern (even though no study has been performed to establish the specificity of this approach).[34–36]

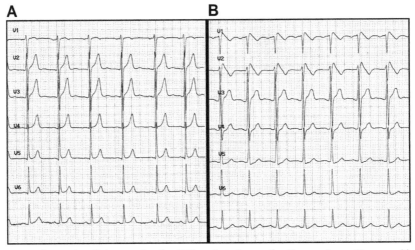

Fig. 2. Ajmaline test during familial screening for BS in a first-degree family member with normal basal ECG (precordial leads). (*A*) Basal ECG. (*B*) After infusion of 1 mg/kg of ajmaline, a type I ECG is observed in leads V_{1-2}.

Table 2
Drugs used to unmask Brugada syndrome

Drug	Dosage	Route of Administration	Duration of Administration
Ajmaline	1 mg/kg	Intravenous	5 min
Flecainide	2 mg/kg	Intravenous	10 min
	400 mg	Orally	Single dose
Procainamide	10 mg/kg	Intravenous	10 min
Pilsicaine	1 mg/kg	Intravenous	10 min

Other techniques have been suggested as diagnostic tools, such as the "full stomach test,"[37] but currently are not being used for this purpose in clinical settings.

DIFFERENTIAL DIAGNOSIS AND ECG MODULATING FACTORS

Many conditions may develop ST-segment elevation in the right precordial leads, mimicking the BS ECG pattern. This group of diseases and ECG abnormalities are not related to BS, and should be carefully ruled out before diagnosing the disease (**Fig. 4**).

Exposure to some drugs and ionic imbalance may also produce a Brugada-like ST-segment elevation. The latter group of circumstances may in fact represent a genetic predisposition to BS,[38] because they exaggerate the ionic imbalance during phase one of the cardiac AP, characteristic of the disease (see later section on "Cellular and ionic mechanisms underlying BS phenotype"; **Fig. 4**).

Fever also modulates the phenotype and risk of arrhythmias in BS patients. Some SCN5A mutations show an accentuation of the inactivation of Na+ channel as temperature rises, and concordantly, fever may elicit a type I ECG pattern and has been identified as a trigger for ventricular arrhythmias.[39–43]

CELLULAR AND IONIC MECHANISMS UNDERLYING BS PHENOTYPE

Under normal conditions, the morphology of the phase one of the action potential (AP) is due to the interaction of two ionic currents: the K+ transient outward current (Ito), which leads to the development of the notch in phase 1 of the AP, and the inward Ca^{+2} current, which is responsible for the dome of the AP during the end of phase 1. Even if the notch in phase 1 is more accentuated in the epicardial cells, the dome is homogeneous through the cells of the different myocardial layers, and no transmural voltage gradients exists during

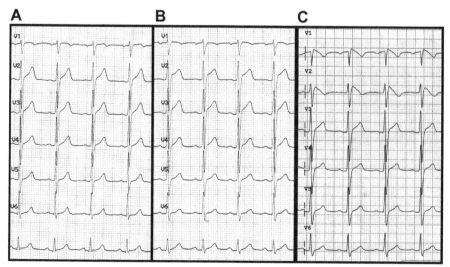

Fig. 3. Pharmacologic challenge with class IA antiarrhythmic drugs during family screening for BS in a first-degree family member with a normal basal ECG (precordial leads). (*A*) Basal ECG. (*B*) Infusion of flecainide, 2 mg/kg, does not unravel a type I ECG pattern. (*C*) Diagnostic ECG pattern in the right precordial leads after ajmaline test.

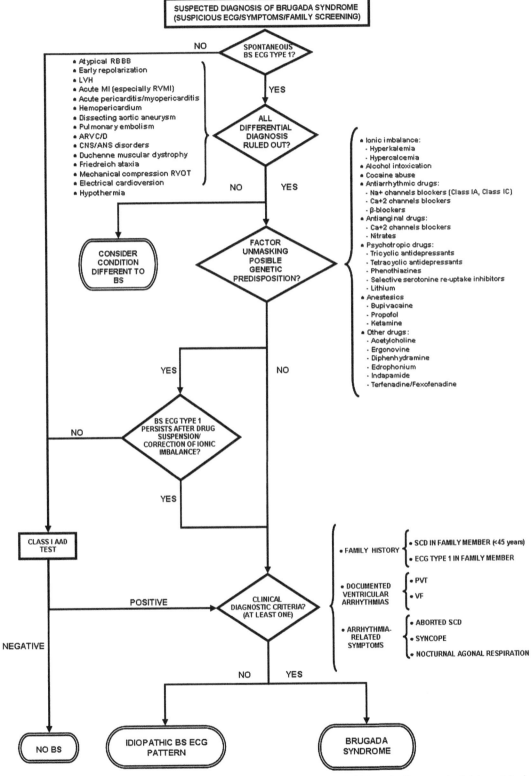

Fig. 4. Diagnostic algorithm for BS. ANS, autonomic nervous system; ARVC/M, arrhythmogenic right ventricular cardiomyopathy/dysplasia; CNS, central nervous system; LVH, left ventricular hypertrophy; MI, myocardial infarction; RBBB, right ventricular bundle branch block; RVMI, right ventricular myocardial infarction; RVOT, right ventricular outflow tract; SCD, sudden cardiac death.

the plateau of the AP, thus the ST-segment is isoelectric.

The ECG manifestations of BS (J point and ST-segment elevation) and the increased risk for ventricular arrhythmias are direct consequences of a shift in balance of the ionic currents active during the end of phase 1 of the AP (decrease of inward positive currents [ie, Na^+ and Ca^{+2}] or increase of outward positive currents [ie, Ito or the glibenclamide-sensitive K_{ATP} potassium current mediated by the Kir6.1 channel]), resulting in an accentuation of the AP notch. This process leads to an elevation of the ST-segment with saddleback appearance, while repolarization of the epicardial cells precedes that of M and endocardial cells and is followed by a positive T wave, and eventually loss-of-dome of the AP, mainly in the right ventricular epicardium, where the Ito is prominent. At this point, the ST-segment elevation will be higher and the morphology will adopt a coved appearance, followed by a negative T wave, secondary to a reversion of the direction of repolarization (from endocardium to epicardium, as the AP in epicardium is prolonged).

The loss-of-dome of the AP at different degrees in the epicardium, the prolonged repolarization phase in the epicardium, and the maintenance of the normal or almost-normal AP profile in the endocardium generate a remarkable dispersion of repolarization within the epicardium and transmurally. Propagation of the AP dome from sites where it is maintained to sites where it is abolished cause local re-excitation (referred to as *phase 2 reentry*), resulting in ventricular extrasystoles originating in the epicardium. These extrasystoles may trigger episodes of PVT/VF in BS (**Fig. 5**). Evidence that these are the mechanisms that underlie the ECG pattern and generate the arrhythmogenic substrate have been published by many authors (in animal models and in humans).[26,44–47]

Differences in expression and density of Ito current between men and women (density of the Ito current is higher in men than in women[48,49]) and hormonal influence[50–53] (estrogens inhibit Ito expression and trafficking, whereas testosterone increases slow potassium currents [IKs]) are the two main hypotheses explaining the predominance of Brugada phenotype among men.

BRUGADA SYNDROME VERSUS IDIOPATHIC BRUGADA ECG PATTERN: ARE THEY REALLY DIFFERENT?

Once a type I ECG is found in right precordial leads, and other conditions that may account for it are excluded, clinical data should be sought to support the diagnosis of BS. The three kinds of diagnostic clinical criteria are listed in **Box 1**.

BS is definitively diagnosed in patients presenting with a type I ECG (either spontaneously or elicited by class I AADs) and at least one of the clinical criteria. The first consensus stated that if a type I ECG was observed in the absence of any clinical criteria, it should be referred to as *idiopathic Brugada ECG pattern* and not BS. Recent data from the authors' group[54,55] suggest that even patients presenting with the diagnostic ECG pattern (in the absence of any clinical criteria) may be at risk of sudden cardiac death. These facts, together with the increasing role of genetic testing in diagnosing the condition, highlight the need for a review of diagnostic criteria for BS. **Fig. 4** shows a proposed diagnostic algorithm.

BS patients may also complain of palpitations because they have a high incidence of supraventricular arrhythmias (up to 30% according to some series).[56–59] Although most of them are atrial fibrillation (**Fig. 6**), other types of supraventricular arrhythmias have also been reported. Furthermore, one study associated the history of supraventricular arrhythmias in BS patients with a higher incidence of ventricular arrhythmias and appropriate shocks, suggesting a more severe stage of the disease.[59] Some BS patients also present with prolonged sinus node recovery and sinoatrial conduction times, slowed atrial conduction, and atrial standstill.[60,61]

PROGNOSIS AND RISK STRATIFICATION

After BS is diagnosed, the next step is risk stratification, being its main objective the accurate identification and treatment of individuals at high risk for sudden cardiac death. To date, some markers of high risk in BS patients have been clearly identified and accepted by all groups, but the issue of risk stratification for asymptomatic BS patients remains controversial.

Survivors of SCD are at high risk of recurrence or life-threatening arrhythmias (17%–62% at 48–84 months follow-up according to different series), and therefore should receive an implantable cardioverter-defibrillator (ICD) for secondary prevention (class I indication).[7–12,62]

Syncope is also a marker of high risk for presenting ventricular arrhythmias (recurrence rate, 6%–19% at 24–39 months follow-up in different series), and patients should receive an ICD, after noncardiac causes of this symptom have been carefully ruled out (class I indication).[7–12,62]

Placement of an ICD is reasonable in patients with BS and documented ventricular tachycardia (VT) not resulting in aborted sudden cardiac death,

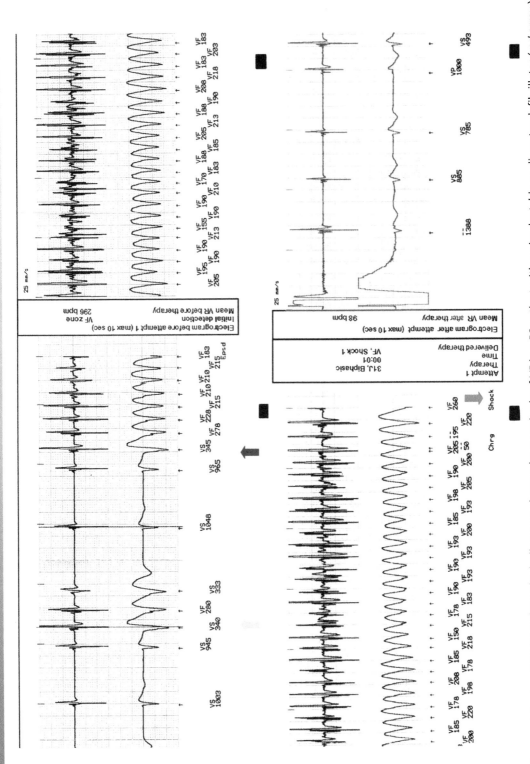

Fig. 5. A nonsustained ventricular tachycardia (*yellow arrow*) precedes an episode of VF in a BS patient with an implantable cardioverter-defibrillator (*red arrow*). The device effectively detects and treats the VF episode with a 31 J shock (*green arrow*).

regardless of their symptomatic status (class IIa indication).[62]

A recent study by Giustetto and colleagues[11] stated that patients with BS and syncope had a similar rate of arrhythmic events during follow-up, irrespective of whether syncopal events were preceded by prodromes (7.4% vs 9.7%, respectively; $P = .9$), concluding that syncope in patients with BS is always a sign of bad prognosis (even if syncope is suspected to be of vasovagal origin based on clinic profile). The value of tilt test in this group could not be established, because none of the patients undergoing tilt test presented arrhythmic events in the follow-up. Because of the limited information in this regard, it is probably too early to recommend protection with an ICD for all patients with any type of syncope.

Spontaneous ECG type I has been identified as an independent predictor of ventricular arrhythmias in multivariate analysis of the largest cohort of BS patients published to date[12] (hazard ratio, 1.8; 95% CI, 1.03–3.33; $P = .04$) and in most other series. Clinical monitoring of ECG is recommended to detect spontaneous type I ECG in BS patients with diagnostic ECG pattern only after pharmacologic challenge with class I AADs, with or without previous symptoms (class IIa indication).[62]

Men showed a tendency to develop more arrhythmic events than women in some series, but the difference did not reach statistical significance.[12,54]

The risk of lethal or near-lethal arrhythmic episodes among previously asymptomatic patients with BS varies according to the series. Brugada and colleagues[9] reported an 8% recurrence rate at 33 ± 39 months of follow-up (HR, 2.5; 95% CI = 1.2–5.3; $P = .017$); Priori and

colleagues[7] reported a 6% recurrence rate at 34 ± 44 months of follow-up; whereas Eckardt and colleagues[10] and Giustetto and colleagues[11] reported a 1% recurrence rate (after 40 ± 50 months and 30 ± 21 months of follow-up, respectively). Finally, Probst and colleagues[12] reported a 1.5% recurrence rate at 31 months of follow-up.

The value of inducibility of sustained ventricular arrhythmias during electrophysiologic study (EPS) as a tool to evaluate arrhythmic risk in BS is still the most controversial topic. Results published by Brugada and colleagues[9] indicate that inducibility during EPS is an independent predictor of cardiac events (hazard ratio, 8.33, 95% CI, 2.8–25; $P = .0001$), and a recent publication by Giustetto and colleagues[11] presented similar results (none of the patients with a negative EPS developed arrhythmic events vs 15% of patients with a positive EPS result during 30 ± 21 months of follow-up), although the remainder of the registries failed to show this.[7,10,12]

The most recent publication on the issue, which is also the largest published series involving BS patients, found that inducibility of sustained ventricular tachyarrhythmias was significantly associated with a shorter time to first arrhythmic event (compared with BS patients not inducible in the EPS) in the univariate analysis (in the global population and in the asymptomatic subgroup), but inducibility did not predict arrhythmic events in the multivariable analysis.[12]

Several proposed reasons may account for this and other differences among the registries, including differences in inclusion criteria, stimulation protocols, and statistical analysis methods. For cases with low event rates and short follow-up in patients with diseases associated with lifelong risk of arrhythmias, drawing definitive conclusions about the predictive value of any test is difficult, and the role of EPS in risk stratification for patients with BS probably will remain undefined or controversial until prospective data are obtained in patients studied with a uniform protocol in a large population with adequate and, especially, long follow-up. Current guidelines consider EPS for risk stratification a class IIb indication in asymptomatic BS patients with spontaneous type I ECG.[62]

Family history of sudden cardiac death has not been identified as a reliable marker of high-risk in patients affected by Brugada syndrome.[9,12]

In all published series, no difference in arrhythmic events was seen when dividing patients according to the presence or absence of *SCN5A* genetic mutations. A recent study involving 147 BS patients with *SCN5A* identified mutations showed a significantly higher rate of syncope among patients with *SCN5A* truncation mutations (caused by

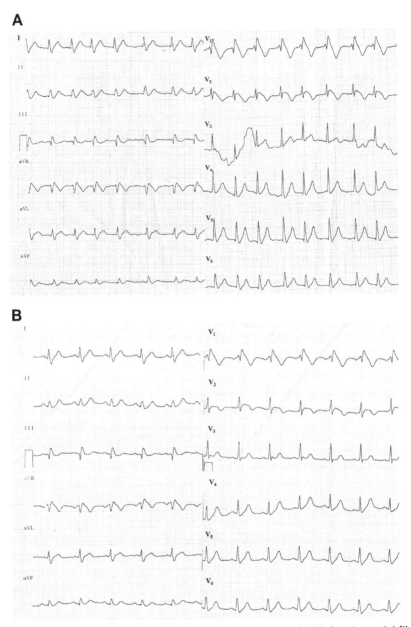

Fig. 6. Patient diagnosed with BS complaining of palpitations. (*A*) A 12-lead ECG showing atrial fibrillation at 90 bpm and a type I ECG pattern of BS in leads V_1 and V_2. (*B*) A 12-lead ECG of the same patient, after reversion to sinus rhythm.

a premature stop codon) and those with *SCN5A* missense mutations resulting in a decrease of more than 90% of the nonfunctional Na^+ channels than among those with *SCN5A* missense mutations that produce a lesser decrease of Na current ($\leq$90%). The investigators could not show a higher rate of more serious arrhythmic events (SCD or VF) in patients with mutations encoding nonfunctional Na^+ channels. The first two groups of patients also presented with longer PR intervals in the basal

ECG, and showed a greater increase of PR and QRS intervals after the class I AAD test. This study was the first to propose using genetic data in risk stratification for BS.[63]

The recent finding that common polymorphisms located in *SCN5A* may modulate the effect of mutations causing BS,[64,65] resulting in a counter-balance of its deleterious consequences with improvement of the BS phenotype, presents the possibility of identifying polymorphisms as risk stratification tools, and suggests that polymorphisms may be possible targets for therapeutic interventions.

Fig. 7 shows a proposed risk stratification scheme and recommendations for ICD in BS patients.

POSTULATED NONINVASIVE MARKERS OF ARRHYTHMIC RISK IN BS

In an effort to solve the complex issue of risk stratification in BS, several noninvasive methods have been postulated as markers of arrhythmic events among these patients. A decreased nocturnal standard deviation of the 5 minutes averaged NN intervals (SDANN) measured in Holter recordings[66]; an S wave width in V_1 of 80 miliseconds (ms) or greater and ST-segment elevation in V_2 of

0.18 mV or greater[67]; spontaneous changes in ST segment,[68] a corrected QT interval (QTc) higher than 460 ms in V_2, and prolonged T peak—T end interval and dispersion[69]; the "aVR sign" (R wave $\geq$ 0.3 mV or R/q $\geq$ 0.75 in lead aVR)[70]; prolonged QRS duration in precordial leads (R—J interval in $V_2 \geq$ 90 ms and QRS $\geq$ 90 ms in V_6; QRS $\geq$ 120 ms in V_2)[71]; and, recently, even an indicator of interventricular mechanical dyssynchrony was found to be associated with high risk of fatal or near-fatal arrhythmias in BS.[72] The usefulness of late potentials (LP) assessed by signal-averaged ECG (SAECG) as a marker of high risk was extensively studied by various groups,[30,68,73,74] and a recent prospective study showed that positive LP was an independent marker of high risk in BS patients, with a hazard ratio of 10.9 (95% CI, 1.1—104.3; P = .038), sensitivity of 95.7%, specificity of

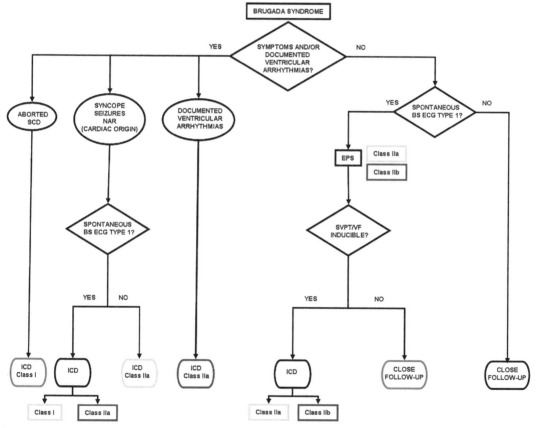

Fig. 7. Proposed risk stratification scheme and recommendations of ICD in BS patients. Yellow boxes denote recommendations from the Second Consensus Conference on Brugada syndrome[6]; red boxes denote recommendations from the ACC/AHA/ESC 2006 Guidelines for Management of Patients With Ventricular Arrhythmias and the Prevention of Sudden Cardiac Death[62]; and green boxes denote recommendations in agreement with both the Brugada Syndrome: Report of the Second Consensus Conference[6] and the ACC/AHA/ESC 2006 Guidelines for Management of Patients With Ventricular Arrhythmias and the Prevention of Sudden Cardiac Death.[62] AAD, antiarrhythmic drugs; Class I: clear evidence that the treatment/intervention is useful or effective; Class II: conflicting evidence about usefulness or efficacy; Class IIa: weight of evidence favors usefulness or efficacy; Class IIb: usefulness or efficacy less well established; NAR, nocturnal agonal respiration; SCD, sudden cardiac death.

65%, positive predictive value of 75.9%, negative predictive value of 92.9%, and predictive accuracy 81.4%.[75] However, before including any of these markers in the BS risk stratification scheme, more prospective studies are needed, including more patients and a longer follow-up.

In conclusion, risk stratification is really the most controversial issue so far. The literature reflects two types of series: those with almost no events during follow-up, and in which the lack of events obviously confers a negative value to any studied factor, and others that have a reasonable number of events during follow-up and have studied different factors that have shown to be of value for risk stratification. The discussion is not which factor is more efficient to stratify patients, but rather why such a big and unexplained difference exists among series. Certainly some new international consensus must be performed, basically on how to diagnose BS based on the new and updated studies that have been published since the last one.

THERAPEUTIC OPTIONS AND RECOMMENDATIONS FOR BS PATIENTS
ICD

To date, the only proven effective therapeutic strategy for preventing sudden cardiac death in BS patients is the ICD. ICDs are not free from several disadvantages, especially in this group of patients who share a particular profile, including active and young individuals, facing a long-lasting coexistence with the device and multiple device replacements, and long life expectation (especially since device implantation). Some series have reported low rates of appropriate shocks (8%–15%, median follow-up 45 months; annual appropriate discharge rate, 2.6%) and high rates of complications, mainly inappropriate shocks (20%–36% at 21–47 months follow-up). In many series, inappropriate shocks greatly exceeded (2 to 2.5 times) the rate of appropriate shocks.[76–78]

Inappropriate shocks (shocks delivered by the ICD for a non–VT/VF rhythm) are caused by various situations, frequently occurring in patients with BS: sinus tachycardia (because most patients are very young and active), atrial tachyarrhythmias, and lead damage, causing sensing of artifacts or myopotentials. Careful programming of the ICD helps avoid inappropriate shocks, including programming only one therapy zone (for VF) at a high rate cutoff (250 beats per minute [bpm] minus patient age in years; or heart rate > 210–220 bpm)[79] and increasing the detection window (ie, programming long detection intervals through increasing the number of intervals to detect VF to 18 of 24,[80,81] with the goal to avoid shocking a nonsustained tachycardia).

Other measures to avoid ICD complications involve emphasizing the absolute contraindication of competitive sports and limitations of recreational sports,[82] especially those such as rowing, swimming, and weightlifting (which are associated with a higher risk for lead damage); favoring the use of one-lead systems (which have been shown to have a lower rate of complications); and treating supraventricular arrhythmias, including radiofrequency catheter ablation (RFCA).

PHARMACOLOGIC TREATMENT IN BS

To rebalance the ionic currents affected in BS during the cardiac AP, drugs that inhibit the Ito current or increase the Na^+ and Ca^{+2} currents have been tested in BS.

Isoproterenol (which increases the ICa current) has been useful for treating electrical storm in BS (class IIa indication).[62] Quinidine, a class Ia AAD with Ito and I-Kr blocker effects, has been shown to prevent induction of VF and suppress spontaneous ventricular arrhythmias in a clinical setting, and is currently being used in patients with ICD and multiple shocks; cases in which ICD implantation is contraindicated; and for treating supraventricular arrhythmias. Experts have also suggested that it could be useful in children with BS or as a bridge or alternative to ICD. However, it also has been had a high rate of secondary effects.[83–86] Quinidine has proved useful for treating electrical storm in BS patients,[87,88] and its use in this context is a class IIb indication.[62]

Dysopiramide[89] and orciprenaline[88,90] have also been shown to be useful in electrical storm in some reports. Other drugs being evaluated for BS are tedisamile (a pure Ito blocker[91,92]), phosphodiesterase III inhibitors (cilostazol[93,94]), and dimethyl lithospermate B.[95]

RFCA IN BS: WILL IT HAVE A REAL CLINICAL APPLICATION?

After a study of a group of patients with high-risk BS who underwent ICD implantation showed that 67% of the VF events were triggered by ventricular ectopy, identical in morphology to frequently found ventricular premature beats (VPBs),[96] RFCA of ventricular ectopy was postulated as a therapeutic approach in BS patients. In three patients with high-risk BS implanted with an ICD, Haissagüerre and colleagues[97] observed clinical episodes of PVT/VF during follow-up, with ambulatory monitoring or stored electrograms of the

ICD showing that VPBs triggered VF. VPBs were monomorphic (two originating in the right ventricular outflow track [RVOT] and one with left BBB and superior axis). During EPS, RFCA was applied at the site of earliest electrogram relative to the onset of the ectopic QRS complex. In the acute setting, inducibility of VF was modified by RFCA in two patients (converting them to noninducible), and during a mean follow-up of 7 ± 6 months no recurrence of VF, syncope, or sudden cardiac death was observed.

Darmon and colleagues[98] also report on a very symptomatic BS patient, with multiple episodes of VT/VF adequately treated with ICD, who was refractory to quinidine. This patient also presented with isolated monomorphic VPBs originating in the RVOT (of myocardial origin, given the fact that VPBs electrograms were not preceded by Purkinje potential). The patient underwent two RFCA procedures (the first for VPB arising from the RVOT, and the second to the RVOT lateral and septal walls), and after 6 months of follow-up did not experience any sustained ventricular arrhythmia.

Nakagawa and colleagues[99] present a similar case report involving a 41-year-old patient with BS with electrical storms suppressed by isoproterenol infusion, recurrent after suspension of that drug, and refractory to quinidine and cilostazol. Because VPBs initiating VF always presented identical morphology and were frequent (posterior portion of the RVOT lateral wall), RFCA was performed. After 29 months of follow-up the patient had experienced no sustained ventricular arrhythmias.

An elegant study performed in 2009 by Morita and colleagues[100] examined the effect of RFCA on 17 arterially perfused canine right ventricular preparations, in which a model of BS was pharmacologically induced (using pinacidil and pilsicaine). They performed RFCA at the earliest activation site of premature ventricular complexes in epicardium or endocardium. At baseline, the AP duration was shorter in the epicardium, no AP duration heterogeneity occurred within the epicardium, and the notch in phase one of AP was deeper in this myocardial layer. Once BS was pharmacologically induced, the epicardium showed AP dispersion heterogeneity, and the notch in phase one of the AP was deeper in the areas where the AP was shorter. After RFCA, the AP dispersion heterogeneity was still present, but the disconnection of areas with long and short AP eliminated ventricular arrhythmia.

Suitable candidates for this approach are very symptomatic patients (multiple episodes of VF/appropriated shocks) presenting with frequent VPBs with a mapable morphology who are refractory to pharmacologic treatment. From the published data, the optimal time for RFCA is the perielectrical storm period (because VPBs are more frequent then). The authors, however, despite the fact that they are following up on a large cohort of patients, have not been able to determine an optimal time for RFCA.

OTHER RECOMMENDATIONS

Patients with BS should be advised to avoid all drugs that may induce a type I ECG or trigger ventricular arrhythmias, and avoid unnecessary use of drugs (because even though a drug has not yet been identified as potentially dangerous for these patients, it is not necessarily safe). The BrugadaDrugs.org Web site provides up-to-date information on this matter.[101]

Because fever may elicit the diagnostic ECG pattern, and has also been recognized as a trigger of ventricular arrhythmias in BS, patients should be encouraged to treat it aggressively. Electrocardiographic monitoring is also recommended in those who have fever.

Patients must contact their cardiologist immediately if they experience syncope, seizures, or nocturnal agonal respiration.

All BS patients must be followed up regularly to monitor the development of symptoms.

Family screening for BS is strongly recommended in first-degree relatives. Genetic testing is recommended if available (to support clinical diagnosis, for early disease detection in other affected family members, and for research purposes).

SUMMARY

After 18 years since its initial description, the scientific knowledge of Brugada syndrome has grown exponentially in many aspects of the disease (genetic and molecular basis, arrhythmogenic mechanisms, clinical course, risk stratification, and treatment). However, substantial controversies remain, especially regarding risk stratification of asymptomatic patients. Given the enormous amount of valuable information collected by many groups since the second consensus was published, current diagnostic criteria, recommended prognostic tools, and treatment must be reviewed. Data emerging from prospective trials will help refine the diagnostic and therapeutic approach to treating patients with BS.

ACKNOWLEDGMENTS

The authors would like to thank David Andreu, BEng, Juan Fernandez-Armenta Pastor, MD, and

Hrvojka M. Zeljko, MD, PhD, for their helpful comments and suggestions during the preparation of figures for this paper.

REFERENCES

1. Brugada P, Brugada J. Right bundle branch block, persistent ST segment elevation and sudden cardiac death: a distinct clinical and electrocardiographic syndrome. A multicenter report. J Am Coll Cardiol 1992;20(6):1391–6.
2. Hermida JS, Lemoine JL, Bou Aoun F, et al. Prevalence of the Brugada syndrome in an apparently healthy population. Eur Heart J 2000;86(1):91–4.
3. Donohue D, Tehrani F, Jamehdor R, et al. The prevalence of Brugada ECG in adult patients in a large university hospital in the western United States. Am Heart Hosp J 2008;6(1):48–50.
4. Sinner MF, Pfeufer A, Perz S, et al. Spontaneous Brugada electrocardiogram patterns are rare in the German general population: results from the KORA study. Europace 2009;11(10):1338–44.
5. Miyasaka Y, Tsuji H, Yamada K, et al. Prevalence and mortality of the Brugada-type electrocardiogram in one city in Japan. J Am Coll Cardiol 2001;38(3):771–4.
6. Antzelevitch C, Brugada P, Borggrefe M, et al. Brugada syndrome: report of the Second Consensus Conference: endorsed by the Heart Rhythm Society and the European Heart Rhythm Association. Circulation 2005;111(5):659–70.
7. Priori SG, Napolitano C, Gasparini M, et al. Natural history of Brugada syndrome: insights for risk stratification and management. Circulation 2002;105(11):1342–7.
8. Brugada J, Brugada R, Antzelevitch C, et al. Long-term follow-up of individuals with the electrocardiographic pattern of right bundle-branch block and ST-segment elevation in precordial leads V1 to V3. Circulation 2002;105(1):73–8.
9. Brugada J, Brugada R, Brugada P. Determinants of sudden cardiac death in individuals with the electrocardiographic pattern of Brugada syndrome and no previous cardiac arrest. Circulation 2003;108(25):3092–6.
10. Eckardt L, Probst V, Smits JP, et al. Long-term prognosis of individuals with right precordial st-segment-elevation Brugada syndrome. Circulation 2005;111(3):257–63.
11. Giustetto C, Drago S, Demarchi PG, et al. Risk stratification of the patients with Brugada type electrocardiogram: a community-based prospective study. Europace 2009;11(4):507–13.
12. Probst V, Veltmann C, Eckardt L, et al. Long-term prognosis of patients diagnosed with Brugada syndrome: results from the FINGER Brugada syndrome registry. Circulation 2010;121(5):635–43.
13. Vatta M, Dumaine R, Varghese G, et al. Genetic and biophysical basis of sudden unexplained nocturnal death syndrome (SUNDS), a disease allelic to Brugada syndrome. Hum Mol Genet 2002;11(3):337–45.
14. Skinner JR, Chung SK, Montgomery D, et al. Near-miss SIDS due to Brugada syndrome. Arch Dis Child 2005;90(5):528–9.
15. Dettmeyer RB, Kandolf R. Cardiomyopathies—misdiagnosed as Sudden Infant Death Syndrome (SIDS). Forensic Sci Int 2010;194(1–3):e21–4.
16. Chen Q, Kirsch GE, Zhang D, et al. Genetic basis and molecular mechanism for idiopathic ventricular fibrillation. Nature 1998;392(6673):293–6.
17. Kapplinger JD, Tester DJ, Alders M, et al. An international compendium of mutations in the SCN5A-encoded cardiac sodium channel in patients referred for Brugada syndrome genetic testing. Heart Rhythm 2010;7(1):33–46.
18. London B, Michalec M, Mehdi H, et al. Mutation in glycerol-3-phosphate dehydrogenase 1-like gene (GPD1-L) decreases cardiac Na+ current and causes inherited arrhythmias. Circulation 2007;116(20):2260–8.
19. Antzelevitch C, Pollevick GD, Cordeiro JM, et al. Loss-of-function mutations in the cardiac calcium channel underlie a new clinical entity characterized by ST-segment elevation, short QT intervals, and sudden cardiac death. Circulation 2007;115(4):442–9.
20. Delpon E, Cordeiro JM, Nunez L, et al. Functional effects of KCNE3 mutation and its role in the development of Brugada syndrome. Circ Arrhythm Electrophysiol 2008;1(3):209–18.
21. Watanabe H, Koopmann TT, Le SS, et al. Sodium channel beta1 subunit mutations associated with Brugada syndrome and cardiac conduction disease in humans. J Clin Invest 2008;118(6):2260–8.
22. Hu D, Barajas-Martinez H, Burashnikov E, et al. A mutation in the beta 3 subunit of the cardiac sodium channel associated with Brugada ECG phenotype. Circ Cardiovasc Genet 2009;2(3):270–8.
23. Medeiros-Domingo A, Tan BH, Crotti L, et al. Gain-of-function mutation, S422L, in the KCNJ8-encoded cardiac K ATP channel Kir6.1 as a pathogenic substrate for J wave syndromes. Heart Rhythm 2010;7(10):1466–71.
24. Wilde A, Antzelevitch C, Borggrefe M, et al. Proposed diagnostic criteria for the Brugada syndrome: consensus report. Circulation 2002;106:2514–9.
25. Sarkozy A, Chierchia GB, Paparella G, et al. Inferior and lateral electrocardiographic repolarization abnormalities in Brugada syndrome. Circ Arrhythm Electrophysiol 2009;2(2):154–61.

26. Gussak I, Antzelevitch C, Bjerregaard P, et al. The Brugada syndrome: clinical, electrophysiologic and genetic aspects. J Am Coll Cardiol 1999; 33(1):5–15.

27. Kasanuki H, Ohnishi S, Ohtuka M, et al. Idiopathic ventricular fibrillation induced with vagal activity in patients without obvious heart disease. Circulation 1997;95(9):2277–85.

28. Richter S, Sarkozy A, Paparella G, et al. Number of electrocardiogram leads displaying the diagnostic coved-type pattern in Brugada syndrome: a diagnostic consensus criterion to be revised. Eur Heart J 2010;31(11):1357–64.

29. Veltmann C, Schimpf R, Echternach C, et al. A prospective study on spontaneous fluctuations between diagnostic and non-diagnostic ECGs in Brugada syndrome: implications for correct phenotyping and risk stratification. Eur Heart J 2006; 27(21):2544–52.

30. Tatsumi H, Takagi M, Nakagawa E, et al. Risk stratification in patients with Brugada syndrome: analysis of daily fluctuations in 12-lead electrocardiogram (ECG) and signal-averaged electrocardiogram (SAECG). J Cardiovasc Electrophysiol 2006;17(7): 705–11.

31. Antzelevitch C. Brugada syndrome. Pacing Clin Electrophysiol 2006;29(10):1130–59.

32. Hong K, Brugada J, Oliva A, et al. Value of electrocardiographic parameters and ajmaline test in the diagnosis of Brugada syndrome caused by SCN5A mutations. Circulation 2004;110(19): 3023–7.

33. Meregalli PG, Ruijter JM, Hofman N, et al. Diagnostic value of flecainide testing in unmasking SCN5A-related Brugada syndrome. J Cardiovasc Electrophysiol 2006;17(8):857–64.

34. Shimizu W, Matsuo K, Takagi M, et al. Body surface distribution and response to drugs of ST segment elevation in Brugada syndrome: clinical implication of eighty-seven-lead body surface potential mapping and its application to twelve-lead electrocardiograms. J Cardiovasc Electrophysiol 2000; 11(4):396–404.

35. Sangwatanaroj S, Prechawat S, Sunsaneewitayakul B, et al. New electrocardiographic leads and the procainamide test for the detection of the Brugada sign in sudden unexplained death syndrome survivors and their relatives. Eur Heart J 2001;22(24):2290–6.

36. Sangwatanaroj S, Prechawat S, Sunsaneewitayakul B, et al. Right ventricular electrocardiographic leads for detection of Brugada syndrome in sudden unexplained death syndrome survivors and their relatives. Clin Cardiol 2001;24(12):776–81.

37. Ikeda T, Abe A, Yusu S, et al. The full stomach test as a novel diagnostic technique for identifying patients at risk of Brugada syndrome. J Cardiovasc Electrophysiol 2006;17(6):602–7.

38. Benito B, Brugada R, Brugada J, et al. Brugada syndrome. Prog Cardiovasc Dis 2008;51(1):1–22.

39. Dumaine R, Towbin JA, Brugada P, et al. Ionic mechanisms responsible for the electrocardiographic phenotype of the Brugada syndrome are temperature dependent. Circ Res 1999;85(9):803–9.

40. Porres JM, Brugada J, Urbistondo V, et al. Fever unmasking the Brugada syndrome. Pacing Clin Electrophysiol 2002;25(11):1646–8.

41. Gonzalez Rebollo JM, Hernandez MA, Garcia A, et al. [Recurrent ventricular fibrillation during a febrile illness in a patient with the Brugada syndrome]. Rev Esp Cardiol 2000;53(5):755–7 [in Spanish].

42. Mok NS, Priori SG, Napolitano C, et al. A newly characterized SCN5A mutation underlying Brugada syndrome unmasked by hyperthermia. J Cardiovasc Electrophysiol 2003;14(4):407–11.

43. Ortega-Carnicer J, Benezet J, Ceres F. Fever-induced ST-segment elevation and T-wave alternans in a patient with Brugada syndrome. Resuscitation 2003;57(3):315–7.

44. Kurita T, Shimizu W, Inagaki M, et al. The electrophysiologic mechanism of ST-segment elevation in Brugada syndrome. J Am Coll Cardiol 2002; 40(2):330–4.

45. Bloch Thomsen PE, Joergensen RM, Kanters JK, et al. Phase 2 reentry in man. Heart Rhythm 2005; 2(8):797–803.

46. Antzelevitch C. In vivo human demonstration of phase 2 reentry. Heart Rhythm 2005;2(8):804–6.

47. Yan GX, Antzelevitch C. Cellular basis for the Brugada syndrome and other mechanisms of arrhythmogenesis associated with ST-segment elevation. Circulation 1999;100(15):1660–6.

48. Di Diego JM, Cordeiro JM, Goodrow RJ, et al. Ionic and cellular basis for the predominance of the Brugada syndrome phenotype in males. Circulation 2002;106(15):2004–11.

49. Verkerk AO, Wilders R, de GW, et al. Cellular basis of sex disparities in human cardiac electrophysiology. Acta Physiol (Oxf) 2006;187(4): 459–77.

50. Matsuo K, Akahoshi M, Seto S, et al. Disappearance of the Brugada-type electrocardiogram after surgical castration: a role for testosterone and an explanation for the male preponderance. Pacing Clin Electrophysiol 2003;26(7 Pt 1): 1551–3.

51. Shimizu W, Matsuo K, Kokubo Y, et al. Sex hormone and gender difference—role of testosterone on male predominance in Brugada syndrome. J Cardiovasc Electrophysiol 2007;18(4):415–21.

52. Song M, Helguera G, Eghbali M, et al. Remodeling of Kv4.3 potassium channel gene expression under the control of sex hormones. J Biol Chem 2001;276(34):31883–90.

53. Bai CX, Kurokawa J, Tamagawa M, et al. Nontran-scriptional regulation of cardiac repolarization currents by testosterone. Circulation 2005; 112(12):1701–10.

54. Benito B, Sarkozy A, Mont L, et al. Gender differences in clinical manifestations of Brugada syndrome. J Am Coll Cardiol 2008;52(19):1567–73.

55. van den Berg MP, de Boer RA, van Tintelen JP. Brugada syndrome or Brugada electrocardiogram? J Am Coll Cardiol 2009;53(17):1569–70.

56. Eckardt L, Kirchhof P, Loh P, et al. Brugada syndrome and supraventricular tachyarrhythmias: a novel association? J Cardiovasc Electrophysiol 2001;12(6):680–5.

57. Eckardt L, Kirchhof P, Johna R, et al. Wolff-Parkinson-White syndrome associated with Brugada syndrome. Pacing Clin Electrophysiol 2001;24(9 Pt 1):1423–4.

58. Morita H, Kusano-Fukushima K, Nagase S, et al. Atrial fibrillation and atrial vulnerability in patients with Brugada syndrome. J Am Coll Cardiol 2002; 40(8):1437–44.

59. Bordachar P, Reuter S, Garrigue S, et al. Incidence, clinical implications and prognosis of atrial arrhythmias in Brugada syndrome. Eur Heart J 2004; 25(10):879–84.

60. Morita H, Fukushima-Kusano K, Nagase S, et al. Sinus node function in patients with Brugada-type ECG. Circ J 2004;68(5):473–6.

61. Takehara N, Makita N, Kawabe J, et al. A cardiac sodium channel mutation identified in Brugada syndrome associated with atrial standstill. J Intern Med 2004;255(1):137–42.

62. Zipes DP, Camm AJ, Borggrefe M, et al. ACC/AHA/ESC 2006 guidelines for management of patients with ventricular arrhythmias and the prevention of sudden cardiac death: a report of the American College of Cardiology/American Heart Association Task Force and the European Society of Cardiology Committee for Practice Guidelines (Writing Committee to Develop Guidelines for Management of Patients With Ventricular Arrhythmias and the Prevention of Sudden Cardiac Death): developed in collaboration with the European Heart Rhythm Association and the Heart Rhythm Society. Circulation 2006;114(10):e385–484.

63. Meregalli PG, Tan HL, Probst V, et al. Type of SCN5A mutation determines clinical severity and degree of conduction slowing in loss-of-function sodium channelopathies. Heart Rhythm 2009;6(3): 341–8.

64. Poelzing S, Forleo C, Samodell M, et al. SCN5A polymorphism restores trafficking of a Brugada syndrome mutation on a separate gene. Circulation 2006;114(5):368–76.

65. Lizotte E, Junttila MJ, Dube MP, et al. Genetic modulation of Brugada syndrome by a common polymorphism. J Cardiovasc Electrophysiol 2009; 20(10):1137–41.

66. Hermida JS, Leenhardt A, Cauchemez B, et al. Decreased nocturnal standard deviation of averaged NN intervals. An independent marker to identify patients at risk in the Brugada syndrome. Eur Heart J 2003;24(22):2061–9.

67. Atarashi H, Ogawa S. New ECG criteria for high-risk Brugada syndrome. Circ J 2003;67(1):8–10.

68. Ikeda T, Takami M, Sugi K, et al. Noninvasive risk stratification of subjects with a Brugada-type electrocardiogram and no history of cardiac arrest. Ann Noninvasive Electrocardiol 2005;10(4): 396–403.

69. Castro HJ, Antzelevitch C, Tornes BF, et al. Tpeak-Tend and Tpeak-Tend dispersion as risk factors for ventricular tachycardia/ventricular fibrillation in patients with the Brugada syndrome. J Am Coll Cardiol 2006;47(9):1828–34.

70. Babai Bigi MA, Aslani A, Shahrzad S. aVR sign as a risk factor for life-threatening arrhythmic events in patients with Brugada syndrome. Heart Rhythm 2007;4(8):1009–12.

71. Takagi M, Yokoyama Y, Aonuma K, et al. Clinical characteristics and risk stratification in symptomatic and asymptomatic patients with Brugada syndrome: multicenter study in Japan. J Cardiovasc Electrophysiol 2007;18(12):1244–51.

72. Babaee Bigi MA, Moaref AR, Aslani A. Interventricular mechanical dyssynchrony: a novel marker of cardiac events in Brugada syndrome. Heart Rhythm 2008;5(1):79–82.

73. Ikeda T, Sakurada H, Sakabe K, et al. Assessment of noninvasive markers in identifying patients at risk in the Brugada syndrome: insight into risk stratification. J Am Coll Cardiol 2001;37(6):1628–34.

74. Ajiro Y, Hagiwara N, Kasanuki H. Assessment of markers for identifying patients at risk for life-threatening arrhythmic events in Brugada syndrome. J Cardiovasc Electrophysiol 2005; 16(1):45–51.

75. Huang Z, Patel C, Li W, et al. Role of signal-averaged electrocardiograms in arrhythmic risk stratification of patients with Brugada syndrome: a prospective study. Heart Rhythm 2009;6(8): 1156–62.

76. Sacher F, Probst V, Iesaka Y, et al. Outcome after implantation of a cardioverter-defibrillator in patients with Brugada syndrome: a multicenter study. Circulation 2006;114(22):2317–24.

77. Sarkozy A, Boussy T, Kourgiannides G, et al. Long-term follow-up of primary prophylactic implantable cardioverter-defibrillator therapy in Brugada syndrome. Eur Heart J 2007;28(3):334–44.

78. Rosso R, Glick A, Glikson M, et al. Outcome after implantation of cardioverter defibrillator [corrected] in patients with Brugada syndrome: a multicenter

Israeli study (ISRABRU). Isr Med Assoc J 2008; 10(6):435–9.

79. Spragg DD, Berger RD. How to avoid inappropriate shocks. Heart Rhythm 2008;5(5):762–5.

80. Gunderson BD, Abeyratne AI, Olson WH, et al. Effect of programmed number of intervals to detect ventricular fibrillation on implantable cardioverter-defibrillator aborted and unnecessary shocks. Pacing Clin Electrophysiol 2007;30(2):157–65.

81. Wathen MS, DeGroot PJ, Sweeney MO, et al. Prospective randomized multicenter trial of empirical antitachycardia pacing versus shocks for spontaneous rapid ventricular tachycardia in patients with implantable cardioverter-defibrillators: pacing fast ventricular tachycardia reduces shock therapies (PainFREE Rx II) trial results. Circulation 2004; 110(17):2591–6.

82. Heidbuchel H, Corrado D, Biffi A, et al. Recommendations for participation in leisure-time physical activity and competitive sports of patients with arrhythmias and potentially arrhythmogenic conditions. Part II: ventricular arrhythmias, channelopathies and implantable defibrillators. Eur J Cardiovasc Prev Rehabil 2006;13(5):676–86.

83. Belhassen B, Viskin S, Fish R, et al. Effects of electrophysiologic-guided therapy with Class IA antiarrhythmic drugs on the long-term outcome of patients with idiopathic ventricular fibrillation with or without the Brugada syndrome. J Cardiovasc Electrophysiol 1999;10(10):1301–12.

84. Belhassen B, Glick A, Viskin S. Efficacy of quinidine in high-risk patients with Brugada syndrome. Circulation 2004;110(13):1731–7.

85. Hermida JS, Denjoy I, Clerc J, et al. Hydroquinidine therapy in Brugada syndrome. J Am Coll Cardiol 2004;43(10):1853–60.

86. Belhassen B, Glick A, Viskin S. Excellent long-term reproducibility of the electrophysiologic efficacy of quinidine in patients with idiopathic ventricular fibrillation and Brugada syndrome. Pacing Clin Electrophysiol 2009;32(3):294–301.

87. Maury P, Hocini M, Haissaguerre M. Electrical storms in Brugada syndrome: review of pharmacologic and ablative therapeutic options. Indian Pacing Electrophysiol J 2005;5(1):25–34.

88. Schweizer PA, Becker R, Katus HA, et al. Successful acute and long-term management of electrical storm in Brugada syndrome using orciprenaline and quinine/quinidine. Clin Res Cardiol 2010; 99(7):467–70.

89. Sumi S, Maruyama S, Shiga Y, et al. High efficacy of disopyramide in the management of ventricular fibrillation storms in a patient with Brugada syndrome. Pacing Clin Electrophysiol 2010;33(6): e53–6.

90. Kyriazis K, Bahlmann E, van der SH, et al. Electrical storm in Brugada syndrome successfully treated with orciprenaline; effect of low-dose quinidine on the electrocardiogram. Europace 2009;11(5):665–6.

91. Dukes ID, Morad M. Tedisamil inactivates transient outward K+ current in rat ventricular myocytes. Am J Physiol 1989;257(5 Pt 2):H1746–9.

92. Wettwer E, Himmel HM, Amos GJ, et al. Mechanism of block by tedisamil of transient outward current in human ventricular subepicardial myocytes. Br J Pharmacol 1998;125(4):659–66.

93. Tsuchiya T, Ashikaga K, Honda T, et al. Prevention of ventricular fibrillation by cilostazol, an oral phosphodiesterase inhibitor, in a patient with Brugada syndrome. J Cardiovasc Electrophysiol 2002; 13(7):698–701.

94. Abud A, Bagattin D, Goyeneche R, et al. Failure of cilostazol in the prevention of ventricular fibrillation in a patient with Brugada syndrome. J Cardiovasc Electrophysiol 2006;17(2):210–2.

95. Fish JM, Welchons DR, Kim YS, et al. Dimethyl lithospermate B, an extract of Danshen, suppresses arrhythmogenesis associated with the Brugada syndrome. Circulation 2006; 113(11):1393–400.

96. Kakishita M, Kurita T, Matsuo K, et al. Mode of onset of ventricular fibrillation in patients with Brugada syndrome detected by implantable cardioverter defibrillator therapy. J Am Coll Cardiol 2000;36(5):1646–53.

97. Haissagüerre M, Extramiana F, Hocini M, et al. Mapping and ablation of ventricular fibrillation associated with long-QT and Brugada syndromes. Circulation 2003;108(8):925–8.

98. Darmon JP, Bettouche S, Deswardt P, et al. Radiofrequency ablation of ventricular fibrillation and multiple right and left atrial tachycardia in a patient with Brugada syndrome. J Interv Card Electrophysiol 2004;11(3):205–9.

99. Nakagawa E, Takagi M, Tatsumi H, et al. Successful radiofrequency catheter ablation for electrical storm of ventricular fibrillation in a patient with Brugada syndrome. Circ J 2008;72(6):1025–9.

100. Morita H, Zipes DP, Morita ST, et al. Epicardial ablation eliminates ventricular arrhythmias in an experimental model of Brugada syndrome. Heart Rhythm 2009;6(5):665–71.

101. Postema PG, Wolpert C, Amin AS, et al. Drugs and Brugada syndrome patients: review of the literature, recommendations, and an up-to-date website. Heart Rhythm 2009;6(9):1335–41.

Short QT Syndromes

Fiorenzo Gaita, MD[a,b,*], Carla Giustetto, MD[a,b],
Andrea Mazzanti, MD[a,b]

KEYWORDS

- Short QT syndrome • Sudden death • ICD
- Hydroquinidine

The relationship between the QT interval and cardiac arrhythmias has been recognized for half a century, after it was observed that a long QT interval was associated with an increased susceptibility to polymorphic ventricular tachycardia and sudden cardiac death.[1] Only in the last 2 decades the attention has moved to the opposite condition, that is when the QT interval is abnormally short. In 1993, Algra and colleagues[2] published a retrospective study in which the QT interval of 6693 subjects was measured in 24-hour Holter recordings. It was observed that both a prolonged ($\geq$440 ms) and a shortened (<400 ms) mean corrected QT (QTc) interval were associated with a more than 2-fold risk of sudden death compared with intermediate mean QTc values (400–440 ms).

In 2000, Gussak and colleagues[3] described 1 family (a 17-year-old girl with several episodes of paroxysmal atrial fibrillation [AF], her brother, and their mother) that demonstrated QT and QTc intervals less than 300 ms and an unrelated 37-year-old patient with similar electrocardiographic (ECG) changes, who had died suddenly. Finally, with the study by Gaita and colleagues[4] published in 2003, the short QT syndrome (SQTS) was recognized as a new clinical entity related to familial sudden death, suggesting an autosomal dominant inheritance. Seven affected members of 2 distinct European families were described, and a QT interval less than 280 ms was associated with syncope, palpitations, and sudden cardiac death across several generations. These patients showed QT intervals between 210 and 280 ms (with QTc always <300 ms), very short atrial and ventricular refractory periods ($\leq$160 ms and 150 ms, respectively), and

induction of ventricular fibrillation (VF) in most subjects. Moreover, the short QT was present in all the available ECGs of these patients, with only slight variations at different heart rates. The genetic nature of the disease was confirmed shortly after, with the discovery in rapid succession of gain-of-function mutations in 3 genes: KCNH2,[5] KCNQ1,[6] and KCNJ2.[7] These genes code for different potassium channels located on the cell membrane of the cardiomyocytes. More recently have been identified loss-of-function mutations in 2 genes that encode for the α_1- and β_{2b}- subunits of the L-type calcium channel, CACNA1C and CACNB2b, which are responsible for a mixed phenotype of short QT and Brugada aspect.[8]

ECG

The QT interval varies not only among different individuals in relation to the age and the sex[9] but also in the same subject, according to fluctuations in the heart rate or the autonomic tone or due to external factors, such as the use of certain drugs. It is known that to overcome the rate dependence of the QT interval, different correction formulas have been introduced to report any QT value to a standard comparable with other measurements. All these formulas have some limitations. Bazett's formula[10] was introduced in the 1920s; it is based on few observations and is the most used formula in clinical practice, despite its tendency to underestimate the QT interval at low frequencies and to overestimate it at high heart rates. In the early 1990s, Rautaharju and colleagues[11] investigated the ECGs of 14,379 healthy individuals and

This work received no funding support.
The authors have nothing to disclose.
[a] Cardiology Department, Division of Cardiology, Cardinal Massaia Hospital, C.so Dante, 202, Asti 14100, Italy
[b] Division of Cardiology, University of Turin, San Giovanni Battista Hospital, C.so Bramante, 88/90, Turin 10126, Italy
* Corresponding author. Division of Cardiology, University of Turin, San Giovanni Battista Hospital, C.so Bramante, 88/90, 10126 Turin.
E-mail address: gaitaf@libero.it

established a formula by which the expected QT interval can be calculated for a specific heart rate: QT predicted (QTp) = 65,600/(100 + heart rate). Considering that the values of the QT interval have a Gaussian distribution in the population, the lower limit of the normal QT can be set at 2 standard deviations below the QTp (or QT/QTp ≤88%). More recently, other large population-based studies reporting the distribution of QTc in healthy subjects have been published. The work by Gallagher and colleagues[12] examined the ECGs of 12,500 young adults (90% men, mean age 30 ± 10 years) who underwent a medical examination for reasons of employment. In the study by Funada and colleagues,[13] the sample consisted of people examined in a hospital in Japan and who resulted to be healthy (50% men; mean age 50 ± 20 years). In the study by Kobza and colleagues,[14] a group of more than 40,000 Swiss conscripts were examined (99.6% men; mean age 19 ± 1.4 years). Also, in these studies the QTc has a Gaussian distribution. The normal QT interval is defined as a value included between ± 2 standard deviations from the mean, and consequently, 95% of values are normal, whereas values less than the 2.5 percentile and those greater than the 97.5 percentile are too short and too long, respectively. From the statistical considerations on the general population mentioned earlier and according to the previous formulas, a QTc less than 360 ms in men and less than 370 ms in women is considered abnormally short.

The first patients described by the authors' group with SQTS showed QTc intervals that did not exceed the 300 ms and a QT/QTp maximum of 71% (**Fig. 1**, panel A).[4] With the increase in the number of observations, values of QT up to 320 ms and QTc up to 340 ms were subsequently reported.[15,16] Viskin and colleagues[17] found that more than one-third of men with a history of idiopathic VF had a QTc interval of less than 360 ms. The QTc in the patients with a mixed phenotype (Brugada syndrome and SQTS) and in their affected family members ranged from 330 ms to 360 ms in men and 370 ms in women (QT/QTp <88%).[8]

It is likely that, similarly to what happened for the long QT, the first described cases of SQTS were the ones with the most impressive aspect and a high incidence of malignant ventricular arrhythmias, but also values of QTc less than 360 ms can involve some arrhythmic risk. As suggested by Viskin,[18] it is improbable that a single QTc value can distinguish all cases of SQTS from healthy individuals. Instead, overlapping between "short" and "normal" QT intervals mimics what it is known to exist between "normal" and "long."

In the first observed patients (carriers of the N588 K mutation in KCNH2), T waves seem narrow, tall, peaked, and symmetric; a clear ST segment is absent, and the T wave initiates immediately after the S wave.

However, this is not observed in every patient. In SQT2[6] and in most nongenotyped patients, the T wave is still tall and symmetric, despite being less sharp (see **Fig. 1**, panels B and E). In SQT3,[7] in contrast to the other published cases, the T wave shows an asymmetrical pattern with a rather normal ascending phase, followed by a rapid terminal phase (see **Fig. 1**, panel C). Another distinctive ECG feature of patients with SQTS is the relatively prolonged Tpeak-Tend interval. This interval may indicate an augmented transmural dispersion of repolarization, which was demonstrated by Extramiana and Antzelevitch[19] in an animal model.

A further relevant feature in patients with SQTS is the lack of adaptation of the QT interval to the variations in the heart rate.[4,15,20] In SQTS, the QT interval does not show the physiologic shortening in response to an increasing heart rate, but being very short in basal conditions, it decreases only slightly during effort.[4,15,20] Because the QT interval approaches normal values at high rates, it is advisable that the QT interval should be measured as close as possible to 60 b/min.

Another source of error in reading the ECG originates from the practical difficulties in measuring the QT interval.[21] It is a good practice to measure the QT interval in multiple leads, and in these patients, who typically present T waves of high voltage, choose the lead with the highest T wave (most often V2 or V3).

GENETICS

Between 2004 and 2005, mutations in 3 genes encoding potassium channels were identified, all resulting in an increased activity of the channels. The genetic screening in the first reported families with SQTS and sudden cardiac death led to the identification of 2 different missense mutations, resulting in the same amino acid change (asparagine at codon 588 with a positive charged lysine: N588 K) in the S5-P region of the cardiac I_{Kr} channel, KCNH2 (HERG). In vitro functional studies revealed that the mutations increase the I_{Kr} function, leading to a shortening of the action potential duration and reducing the affinity of the channels to the I_{Kr} blockers.[5] This genetic variant has been defined as SQTS type 1 (SQT1). It is interesting to note that mutations determining a reduced function of I_{Kr} are responsible for long QT syndrome type 2.

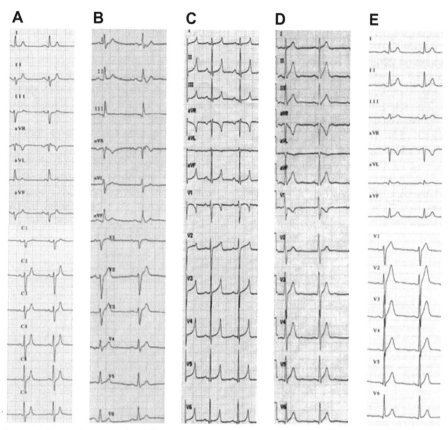

Fig. 1. Each panel shows the ECG of a different genetic variant of SQTS. (*Panel A*) KCNH2 (HERG), SQT1. 31-year-old woman. HR 80 bpm, QT 260 ms, QTc 300 ms, QT/QTp 71%. Note the narrow, sharp, and symmetric T waves. (*Panel B*) KCNQ1, SQT2. 70-year-old man. HR 65 bpm, QT 290 ms, QTc 302 ms, QT/QTp 73%. T waves are still narrow and symmetric but are not peaked (*Adapted from* Bellocq C, Van Ginneken ACG, Bezzina CR, et al. Mutation in the KCNQ1 gene leading to the short QT-interval syndrome. Circulation 2004;109:239). (*Panel C*) KCNJ2, SQT3. 5-year-old child. Respiratory arrhythmia, mean HR 76 bpm, QT 280 ms, QTc 315 ms, QT/QTp 75%. The T waves are noticeably narrow, peaked, and asymmetrical, with a rather normal ascending limb, followed by an extremely rapid terminal phase. (*Courtesy of* Silvia G. Priori, MD, PhD, Molecular Cardiology, Maugeri Foundation, University of Pavia, Italy; New York, University School of Medicine). (*Panel D*) CACNB2b, SQT5. 21-year-old man. HR 71 bpm, QT 300 ms, QTc 327 ms, QT/QTp 78%. Narrow, symmetric, nonpeaked T waves. (*Panel E*) Unknown genotype. 50-year-old man. HR 75 bpm, QT 280 ms, QTc 313 ms, QT/QTp 75%. Narrow, symmetric, non-peaked T waves.

The same N588K mutation in KCNH2[22] was later found in the first family with familial AF, but no history of sudden death was reported by Gussak and colleagues.[3] Some other genetic variants in gene associated with SQT1 have been reported more recently,[23,24] but it has been noted that the finding of sequence variants in any of the genes associated with SQTS is not sufficient to claim that they are the cause of the disease, unless the suspected disease-associated variants show not to be present in a relevant population of controls or that functional analysis is performed to confirm their pathogenetic role.[25,26] Genetic heterogeneity in the SQTS was soon revealed by the findings of 2 different mutations in the KCNQ1 gene that encodes for the slow

component of delayed rectifier I_{Ks} channel; this variety was defined as SQTS type 2 (SQT2). The first observation by Bellocq and colleagues[6] identified a mutation (valine for leucine at codon 307: V307L) in a 70-year-old patient with a QTc of 302 ms and aborted sudden death. The mutation caused a gain of function of I_{Ks}, resulting in a shortening of the action potential duration. The following year, Hong and colleagues[27] identified a second mutation (valine at codon 141 for a methionine: V141 M) in the S1 segment of KCNQ1 in a baby girl born at 38 weeks, after labor induction prompted by bradycardia and irregular rhythm; her ECG revealed AF with slow ventricular response and short QT interval. This variant has been defined as

SQT2; loss-of-function mutations on the same gene are responsible for type 1 long QT syndrome.

Another variant SQT3 was described by Priori and colleagues[7] in 2005 and was associated with a gain of function mutation in the KCNJ2 gene, encoding for the inwardly rectifying channel protein Kir2.1. The 2 affected members of a single family had change from aspartic acid to asparagine at position 172 (D172 N). The functional characterization of the mutation demonstrated a significant increase in the outward I_{K1} current.

On the other hand, a reduced I_{K1} current is involved in the Andersen-Tawil syndrome (long QT syndrome type 7).

In 2007, Antzelevitch and colleagues[8] reported 3 index patients in whom the Brugada syndrome phenotype and a family history for sudden cardiac death were associated with QTc less than or greater than 360 ms (**Fig. 2**, panels A and B). In these 3 cases, a mutation in genes encoding the α_1- or β_{2b}- subunits of the cardiac L-type calcium channel was identified and specifically 2 mutations on CACNA1C (valine for alanine at codon 39: A39 V; arginine for glycine at codon 490: G490R) and a mutation on CACNB2b (substitution of leucine for serine at codon 481: S481L); these variants were called SQT4 and SQT5, respectively (see **Fig. 1**, panel D). The results of patch-clamp

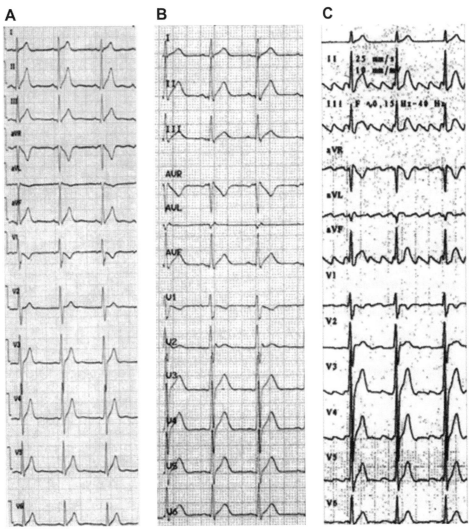

Fig. 2. The panels show 3 different ECGs from the patient with CACNB2b mutation (SQT5) presented in **Fig. 1**, panel D. The first ECG in panel *A* shows the short QT pattern (QT 300 ms, QTc 327 ms, QT/QTp 78%). Panel *B* shows the spontaneous occurrence of a type 3 Brugada pattern in lead V2, QT 300 ms, and QTc 364 ms. Panel *C* shows an episode of atrial flutter with very short FF cycles (170 ms), 4:1 AV conduction, and HR 88 bpm.

experiments indicate that all the mutations cause a major loss of function in calcium channel activity.

At present, however, only a minority of patients (in the authors' experience about 27% of the probands who underwent a genetic screening) received a genetic characterization.

CLINICAL MANIFESTATIONS

SQTS has only been described in the last decade, and in this period less than 60 cases have been reported in the literature worldwide. The authors' database, which derives from the observation of 29 index cases, so far includes 53 subjects (40 men, mean age at observation 30 ± 18 years), 80% of whom had a history of personal or familial sudden death. At the moment of observation, 62% of all the patients were symptomatic. The first clinical presentation was a cardiac arrest in one-third of these cases (17 out of 53). Sudden death was observed in individuals of all ages, mostly children or young adults, including babies in their first months of life, suggesting a possible role for SQTS in some cases of the sudden infant death syndrome. It has not been proved whether a specific trigger can cause a cardiac arrest, as events have occurred both at rest and during exertion or emotion. Syncope was observed as a first clinical presentation in 13% of cases, and the age of its presentation was quite variable, from 8 months to 70 years. It is likely that, as in other channelopathies, syncope is due to episodes of ventricular tachycardia with spontaneous resolution. Episodes of this kind were recorded by the implantable defibrillator (ICD) memory in some cases in asymptomatic patients.

AF has been documented in 17% of patients, also in young individuals; 2 of the first subjects with SQTS were seen at the age of 17 years for episodes of paroxysmal AF[3,4] and 1 case was also documented in utero.[27] Atrial flutter was also documented; FF intervals are typically very short (150–170 ms), as a consequence of the very short atrial refractory periods (see **Fig. 2**, panel C).

DIAGNOSIS

There are some causes of acquired short QT interval that need to be ruled out before considering the diagnosis of SQTS: sinus tachycardia, hyperthermia, electrolyte abnormalities (increased calcium and potassium plasma levels), acidosis, increased vagal tone, and digitalis toxicity.[28]

As in the case of the other channelopathies, structural heart disease is generally absent, as demonstrated by echocardiography and in some cases by cardiac magnetic resonance and autoptic examination.

Holter recordings and stress test document a regular behavior of the heart rate during activity, but only a small variation of the QT interval is observed in relation to the RR cycle,[20] resulting in a reduced slope of the QT-RR relationship as compared with control subjects. This QT-RR relationship is an important element in the diagnosis of SQTS. Because the QT intervals shorten only slightly with the increasing heart rate, QT and QTc tend to approach the normal values at faster heart rates.

At electrophysiologic study, the atrial and ventricular refractory periods are short (140–200 ms at a cycle length between 500 and 600 ms). VF, rarely monomorphic ventricular tachycardia, is induced at programmed ventricular stimulation in about 60% of cases, frequently by mechanical contact during catheter positioning. Also, sustained AF is frequently induced during programmed atrial stimulation. The electrophysiologic study has a role in the diagnosis, confirming the presence of short atrial and ventricular refractory periods, but its role in risk stratification is not clear, as in the authors' experience its sensitivity in reproducing VF in patients with a previous cardiac arrest is about 40%.

RISK STRATIFICATION AND THERAPY

The high incidence of sudden death and the absence of a pharmacologic therapy of proved efficacy in the long term make the ICD the safest choice for the prevention of sudden death in SQTS.[4,15] The ICD is offered not only to patients with a history of cardiac arrest or syncope and to those with induction of VF at electrophysiologic study but also to subjects with a familial history of sudden death, without induced ventricular arrhythmias. A 16-year-old adolescent belonging to the first described families with SQTS and N588 K mutation in KCNH2 experienced an episode of VF, interrupted by shock, shortly after receiving the ICD. This patient had been implanted because of a syncopal episode, which had occurred at the age of 8 months, and for the family history of sudden death over 3 generations, even if no ventricular tachyarrhythmias were induced at electrophysiologic study.[4,29]

The implant of an ICD is not feasible in all patients, and investigators have tried a variety of antiarrhythmic agents in an attempt to correct the electrophysiologic anomalies recognized in patients with SQTS.

Even before the identification of the gain-of-function mutation in KCNH2 in the first described families, the very short QT interval and the symmetric T waves of high amplitude led to the hypothesis of an increased phase 2 or phase 3 potassium currents; for this reason selective I_{Kr} blocking agents were tested (sotalol and ibutilide).[30] These drugs failed to produce an increase in the QT interval in patients with SQT1, and subsequent genetic studies showed that the N588 K mutation in KCNH2 reduced the sensitivity of the channel to sotalol.[5] Among the other drugs, flecainide caused only a slight QT prolongation (mainly because of an increase in the QRS duration) in the 4 patients who tried it.[30] The normalization of the QT interval was instead obtained with hydroquinidine (HQ), which also proved to be effective in lengthening ventricular refractory periods and made the VF non-inducible.[30] Wolpert and colleagues[20] later demonstrated that the N588 K-KCNH2 mutation produced a 5.8-fold decrease in the I_{Kr} channel blocking effect of HQ, in contrast to the 20-fold decrease in the effect of sotalol. The efficacy of HQ was demonstrated in patients with the mutation in KCNH2, whereas in those without, a lower and less homogeneous QTc increment was observed.[15] The efficacy of HQ is also probably due to the blocking effect on other potassium currents (mainly I_{Ks}, I_{K1}, I_{KATP}, and I_{to}). The finding that HQ effectively prolongs the QT interval and prevents ventricular arrhythmias induction is particularly important because patients with SQTS are at risk of sudden death from birth and the implant of an ICD in young children is a complex task for technical reasons (problems related to the small body and heart size, difficult vascular access, and the need for modifications of the implant system during growth) and for the psychological impact of an ICD in younger patients.[31,32] HQ may also be proposed to those patients who refuse the ICD and for the prevention of AF. Other antiarrhythmic drugs that have been tried clinically include propafenone, which suppressed AF but did not prolong the QT interval,[27] and amiodarone, which was successfully used to prevent polymorphic ventricular tachycardia recurrences in a patient with SQTS with an unknown genotype.[33] Disopyramide has been shown to reduce I_{Kr} current blockade only slightly (1.5 fold) in patch-clamp studies on cells expressing the N588 K-KCNH2 mutation[34]; however in the clinical setting the data are limited.[35]

A common complication observed in patients with SQTS treated with an ICD is the occurrence of inappropriate shocks, as the tall and short coupled T waves characteristic in this disorder[4,36] may lead to inappropriate therapies because of double counting of the R and T waves. This complication was seen in 3 of the 5 initially implanted patients.[36] The problem may be prevented looking for an optimal R/T ratio during the implant and with appropriate programming of the other parameters of discrimination. Different algorithms that address T wave oversensing are currently available, but they vary among the manufacturers. A further option is to elevate the maximal ventricular sensitivity for VF detection over the default value of 0.3 mV. However, the value should have been tested during the implant; otherwise VF needs to be reinduced so that continuous detection of VF signals can be verified. Also prophylaxis with HQ may be useful, as it reduces the amplitude of the T waves.

SUMMARY

The SQTS is a recently described genetic arrhythmogenic disorder, characterized by abnormally short QT intervals and a high incidence of sudden death during life, including the first months of life. Therefore, it should also be considered as a possible cause of the sudden infant death syndrome. Often a noticeable family history of cardiac sudden death is present. AF may be observed, also in young individuals. The inheritance is autosomal dominant, with genetic heterogeneity. Gain-of-function mutations in 3 genes encoding potassium channels have been identified, explaining the abbreviated repolarization seen in this condition: KCNH2 encoding I_{Kr} (SQT1), KCNQ1 encoding I_{Ks} (SQT2), and KCNJ2 encoding I_{K1} (SQT3). Some cases present with a double phenotype of SQTS and Brugada syndrome. Loss-of-function mutations in 2 genes encoding the cardiac L-type calcium channel, CACNA1C and CACNB2b, have also been found. At electrophysiologic study, short atrial and ventricular refractory periods are found, and AF and VF are easily induced by programmed electrical stimulation. The outcome of patients with SQTS becomes relatively safe when they are identified and treated. Currently, the suggested therapeutic strategy is the implantation of an ICD in patients with personal or familial history of sudden death. Concern exists for elderly asymptomatic patients and for children. In these categories, pharmacologic treatment with HQ, which has been shown to prolong QT and reduce the inducibility of ventricular arrhythmias, may be proposed.

REFERENCES

1. Jervell A, Lange-Nielsen F. Congenital deaf-mutism, functional heart disease with prolongation of the Q-T interval, and sudden death. Am Heart J 1957;54:59–68.
2. Algra A, Tijssen JGP, Roelandt JRTC, et al. QT interval variables from 24 hour electrocardiography

and the two year risk of sudden death. Br Heart J 1993;70:43–8.

3. Gussak I, Brugada P, Brugada J, et al. Idiopathic short QT interval: a new clinical syndrome. Cardiology 2000;94:99–102.

4. Gaita F, Giustetto C, Bianchi F, et al. Short QT syndrome. A familial cause of sudden death. Circulation 2003;108:965–70.

5. Brugada R, Hong K, Dumaine R, et al. Sudden death associated with short-QT syndrome linked to mutations in HERG. Circulation 2004;109:30–5.

6. Bellocq C, Van Ginneken ACG, Bezzina CR, et al. Mutation in the KCNQ1 gene leading to the short QT-interval syndrome. Circulation 2004;109:2394–7.

7. Priori S, Pandit SV, Rivolta I, et al. A novel form of short QT syndrome (SQT3) is caused by a mutation in the KCNJ2 gene. Circ Res 2005;96:800–7.

8. Antzelevitch C, Pollevick GD, Cordeiro JM, et al. Loss-of function mutations in the cardiac calcium channel underlie a new clinical entity characterized by ST-segment elevation, short QT intervals and sudden cardiac death. Circulation 2007;115:442–9.

9. Surawicz B, Parikh SR. Differences between ventricular repolarization in men and women: description, mechanism and implications. Ann Noninvasive Electrocardiol 2003;8:333–40.

10. Bazett HC. An analysis of time relations of the electrocardiograms. Heart 1920;7:353–70.

11. Rautaharju PM, Zhou SH, Wong S, et al. Sex differences in the evolution of the electrocardiographic QT interval with age. Can J Cardiol 1992;8:690–5.

12. Gallagher MM, Magliano G, Yap YG, et al. Distribution and prognostic significance of QT intervals in the lowest half centile in 12,012 apparently healthy persons. Am J Cardiol 2006;98:933–5.

13. Funada A, Hayashi K, Ino H, et al. Assessment of QT intervals and prevalence of short QT syndrome in Japan. Clin Cardiol 2008;31:270–4.

14. Kobza R, Roos M, Niggli B, et al. Prevalence of long and short QT in a young population of 41,767 predominantly male Swiss conscripts. Heart Rhythm 2009;6:652–7.

15. Giustetto C, Di Monte F, Wolpert C, et al. Short QT syndrome: clinical findings and diagnostic-therapeutic implications. Eur Heart J 2006;27:2440–7.

16. Maury P, Hollington L, Duparc A, et al. Short QT syndrome. Should we push the frontier forward? Heart Rhythm 2005;2:1135–7.

17. Viskin S, Zeltser D, Ish-Shalom M, et al. Is idiopathic ventricular fibrillation a short QT syndrome? Comparison of QT intervals of patients with idiopathic ventricular fibrillation and healthy controls. Heart Rhythm 2004;1:587–91.

18. Viskin S. The QT interval: too long, too short or just right. Heart Rhythm 2009;6:711–5.

19. Extramiana F, Antzelevitch C. Amplified transmural dispersion of repolarization as the basis for arrhythmogenesis in a canine ventricular-wedge model of short-QT syndrome. Circulation 2004;110:3661–6.

20. Wolpert C, Schimpf R, Giustetto C, et al. Further insights into the effect of quinidine in short QT syndrome caused by a mutation in HERG. J Cardiovasc Electrophysiol 2005;16:54–8.

21. Lepeschkin E, Surawicz B. The measurement of the Q-T interval of the electrocardiogram. Circulation 1952;6:378–88.

22. Hong K, Bjerregaard P, Gussak I, et al. Short QT syndrome and atrial fibrillation caused by mutation in KCNH2. J Cardiovasc Electrophysiol 2005;16:394–6.

23. Itoh H, Sakaguchi T, Ashihara T, et al. A novel KCNH2 mutation as a modifier for short QT interval. Int J Cardiol 2009;137:83–5.

24. Redpath CJ, Green MS, Birnie DH, et al. Rapid genetic testing facilitating the diagnosis of short QT syndrome. Can J Cardiol 2009;25:e133–5.

25. Hedley PL, Jørgensen P, Schlamowitz S, et al. The genetic basis of long QT and short QT syndromes: a mutation update. Hum Mutat 2009;30:1486–511.

26. Bezzina CR, Verkerk AO, Busjahn A, et al. A common polymorphism in KCNH2 (HERG) hastens cardiac repolarization. Cardiovasc Res 2003;59:27–36.

27. Hong K, Piper DR, Diaz-Valdecantos A, et al. De novo KCNQ1 mutation responsible for atrial fibrillation and short QT syndrome in utero. Cardiovasc Res 2005;68:433–40.

28. Garberoglio L, Giustetto C, Wolpert C, et al. Is acquired short QT due to digitalis intoxication responsible for malignant ventricular arrhythmias? J Electrocardiol 2007;40:43–6.

29. Schimpf R, Bauersfeld U, Gaita F, et al. Short QT syndrome: successful prevention of sudden cardiac death in an adolescent by implantable cardioverter-defibrillator treatment for primary prophylaxis. Heart Rhythm 2005;2:416–7.

30. Gaita F, Giustetto C, Bianchi F, et al. Short QT syndrome: pharmacological treatment. J Am Coll Cardiol 2004;43:1494–9.

31. Boriani G, Biffi M, Valzania C, et al. Short QT Syndrome and arrhythmogenic cardiac diseases in the young: the challenge of implantable cardioverter-defibrillator therapy for children. Eur Heart J 2006;27:2382–4.

32. Thomas SA, Friedmann E, Kao CW, et al. Quality of life and psychological status of patients with implantable cardioverter defibrillators. Am J Crit Care 2006;15:389–98.

33. Lu LX, Zhou W, Zhang X, et al. Short QT syndrome: a case report and review of literature. Resuscitation 2006;71:115–21.

34. McPate MJ, Duncan RS, Witchel HJ, et al. Disopyramide is an effective inhibitor of mutant HERG K+ channels involved in variant 1 short QT syndrome. J Mol Cell Cardiol 2006;41:563–6.

35. Schimpf R, Veltmann C, Giustetto C, et al. In vivo effects of mutant HERG K+ channel inhibition by disopyramide in patients with a short QT-1 syndrome: a pilot study. J Cardiovasc Electrophysiol 2007;18:1157–60.

36. Schimpf R, Wolpert C, Bianchi F, et al. Congenital short QT syndrome and implantable cardioverter defibrillator treatment: inherent risk for inappropriate shock delivery. J Cardiovasc Electrophysiol 2003; 14:1273–7.

Early Repolarization Disease

Ashok J. Shah, MD[a], Frédéric Sacher, MD[a],
Stéphanie Chatel, PhD[b], Nicolas Derval, MD[a],
Vincent Probst, MD, PhD[c], Philippe Mabo, MD[d],
Xingpeng Liu, MD[a], Shinsuke Miyazaki, MD[a],
Amir S. Jadidi, MD[a], Andrei Forclaz, MD[a], Nick Linton, MD[a],
Olivier Xhaet, MD[a], Daniel Scherr, MD[a], Pierre Jais, MD[a],
Meleze Hocini, MD[a], Jean-Jacques Schott, PhD[b],
Michel Haissaguerre, MD[a,*]

KEYWORDS

- Sudden cardiac death • Cardiac arrhythmia • ECG
- Repolarization disease

Sudden cardiac death (SCD) is defined as an unexpected natural death from a cardiac cause within a short time period, generally less than or equal to 1 hour from the onset of symptoms, in a person without any prior condition that would seem to result in instantaneous fatality. Although such a rapid death process is attributed to cardiac arrhythmia, arrhythmia often represents the final common event in a series of events precipitated by known (95%) or unknown (5%) cardiac disorder.[1] SCD accounts for 700,000 deaths annually in the United States and Europe. Most SCD events (90%) are associated with structurally diseased heart caused by coronary arterial abnormalities, dilated and hypertrophic cardiomyopathies, acquired infiltrative disorders, and valvular or congenital cardiac disorder. Primary electrophysiologic disorders (no identifiable structural cardiac problem) with known (long QT syndrome, Brugada syndrome, catecholaminergic polymorphic ventricular tachycardia, short QT syndrome) or unknown (early repolarization [ER] syndrome, idiopathic ventricular fibrillation [VF]) ion-channel abnormalities are responsible for 10% of SCDs.[2,3]

Electrocardiographic (ECG) ER involving the inferolateral leads, which was labeled benign until recently, is the latest of the primary electrical cardiac diseases discovered to have significantly high prevalence in SCD cases and contribute to increased risk of death from cardioarrhythmic cause.[3,4]

DEFINITION OF ECG ER

ER pattern is a common ECG variant, characterized by J-point elevation manifested either as QRS slurring (at the transition from the QRS segment to the ST segment) or notching (a positive deflection inscribed on terminal S wave), ST-segment elevation with upper concavity and prominent T waves in at least two contiguous leads.[5,6] The J point deflection occurring at the QRS-ST junction (also known as "Osborn wave" or "J wave") was first described in 1938 and is seen in both extracardiac and cardiac conditions, such as hypothermia, hypercalcemia, brain injury, hypervagotonia or spinal cord injury leading to loss of sympathetic tone, vasospastic angina, acute posterior myocardial infarction with occlusion of the left circumflex coronary artery, and Brugada syndrome, besides recently described "early repolarization syndrome."[7–9]

In the study by Haissaguerre and colleagues,[3] cases with ER had at least 0.1 mV J-point elevation manifested as QRS slurring or notching in

Conflict of interest statement: None.
[a] Hôpital Cardiologique du Haut-Lévêque, Université Bordeaux II, 33604 Bordeaux, France
[b] l'institut du thorax - UMR 915, Nantes, France
[c] CHU de Nantes, France
[d] CHU de Rennes, France
* Corresponding author.
E-mail address: michel.haissaguerre@chu-bordeaux.fr

Card Electrophysiol Clin 2 (2010) 559–569
doi:10.1016/j.ccep.2010.09.002

the two contiguous inferior or lateral leads (**Fig. 1**). The leads V1 to V3 were not considered in the definition to exclude Brugada syndrome and arrhythmogenic right ventricular cardiomyopathy. To avoid confusion with the pattern commonly seen in highly trained athletes (J-point elevation + ST elevation in V2–V4), the term "inferolateral J-wave elevation syndrome" is probably more appropriate for the ER associated with VF.

PREVALENCE

The prevalence of ER in the general population varies from under 1% to 13%, depending on the age (predominant in young adults), the race (highest among the black population), and the criterion for J-point elevation (0.05 mV vs 0.1 mV).[3,4,10–12]

Using the same ECG criteria as reported by Haissaguerre and colleagues,[3] Tikkanen and colleagues[4] reported the prevalence of ER as 5.8% in a middle-aged population of 10,864 Finnish people. When one considers J-point elevation greater than or equal to 0.2 mV, the prevalence drops to 0.33% (0.7% in the control group studied by Haïssaguerre and colleagues[3]).

In the patients with documented idiopathic VF and structurally normal heart, the prevalence of ER was 31%.[3] Prevalence rates up to 60% have been reported in smaller studies.[13]

JOURNEY FROM BENIGN ECG PATTERN TO A DISORDER OF CARDIAC ACTION POTENTIAL
ER in the Past: a Benign and Normal ECG Variant

It was a widely and a long-held belief that ER on ECG is not associated with any adversity. It would be interesting to know how this concept evolved and became accepted. The authors examined the literature to answer this question and reviewed the articles that were most frequently cited toward this long-held concept. Most of the literature was found to have been published in a period between the early 1950s and late 1970s.[14–19] As shown in **Table 1**, the literature was comprised of observational studies involving 5 to 75 patients with a follow-up period ranging from 6 months to 26 years. Importantly, most of the studies did not have well-matched control groups because their primary objective was to observe the ECG features of ER and not its long-term follow-up. In addition, most of the patients presented with ER only in the precordial leads. The reason for this observation is unclear, although it was noticed that many illustrated ECG tracings were recorded using a direct writer type ECG machine used commonly in that era. These machines generated a very thick baseline that might have been responsible for masking ER in the limb leads. When these studies are evaluated using current standards, the conclusions drawn from them do not seem to bear a strong impact. However, this long-held concept was reconsolidated by Klatsky and colleagues[5] in 2003 in a study involving 73,088 patients who underwent voluntary health examination including ECG in Oakland, California, between 1983 and 1985. The objective of this study was to observe whether patients with ER were at increased risk of hospitalization for chest pain. The cardiologists then set aside the ECGs that had possible ER plus the next two consecutive ECGs, which served as control. This yielded 2234 ECGs, which were photocopied and reinterpreted by the authors in 2000. Excluding the tracings with missing data and those

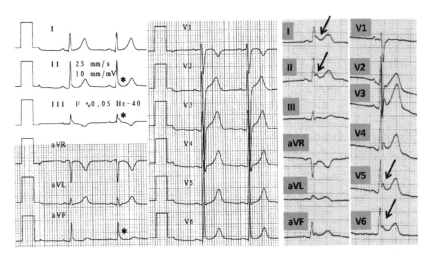

Fig. 1. Different features of J wave elevation as slurring (*asterisks*) or notching (*arrows*) in inferior (*asterisks*) or lateral (*arrows*) in patients with VF.

Table 1
Summary of studies favoring benignancy of early repolarization over 6 to 312 months of follow-up

Author	Year	N	Distribution of ER	Main Findings/Conclusion
Goldman[14]	1953	25	Mid and left precordial leads	2–4 mm J-point elevation in V_{3-6} may occur as a normal variant
Grusin[15]	1954	54	Mainly in precordial leads	ER pattern still presented in 13 but disappeared in 5
Goldman[16]	1960	5	Precordial leads	None developed heart disease and ER remained unchanged
Wasserburger[17]	1961	48	Mainly (77.1%) in precordial leads	ER is a normal RS-T segment elevation variant
Fenichel[18]	1962	75	One or more leads, 62% in lead II	All but two remained free from evident heart disease (angina)
Kambara and Phillips[19]	1976	65	Mainly (85%) in precordial leads	Normal heart size in 46, cardiomegaly in 7, no data in 12

judged as abnormal, finally 2081 ECGs were analyzed including 670 ECGs showing ER. The investigators ascertained medical events during follow-up by computer search of databases through 1998 including hospitalizations and death certificate diagnoses. Outpatient diagnostic data were only available from 1995 to 1999 in 45,528 examinees. The authors concluded that the prevalence of ER in their cohort was 0.9% (670 of 73,088) and the patients with ER were less likely to experience arrhythmias. The overall rate of hospitalization and outpatient visits was not higher than in the control population.

ER in the Current Era: An Electrical Disorder Associated with VF

During the past decade, ER was reported as the only "abnormal" finding in patients diagnosed with idiopathic VF in more than 10 clinical reports from around the globe.[20–22] Meanwhile, the potential arrhythmogenicity of ER was also demonstrated in experimental studies.[23–26] These observations indicated toward a potentially nonbenign nature of ER. More definitive clinical evidence and a turning point in the perception toward ER came in 2007 to 2008, when pioneering work by Haïssaguerre and colleagues[3,27] reported a high prevalence of ER in patients with idiopathic VF. ER was observed in 31% (64 of 206) of idiopathic VF cases versus 5% (21 of 412) of well-matched healthy subjects (P<.001). Furthermore, based on the data from implantable cardioverter-defibrillator, 64 idiopathic VF survivors with ER experienced higher VF

recurrence than 142 VF survivors without ER (41% vs 23%; P = .008). Subsequently, Rosso and colleagues[10] compared the ECGs of 45 idiopathic VF cases with that of 124 age- and gender-matched control subjects and 121 young athletes and found that ER was more common among the patients with VF than among the control subjects (42% vs 13%; P<.001). In another study by Nam and colleagues,[11] baseline ECGs of 11 (57.9%) out of 19 patients with VF showed ER in contrast to 3.3% of 1395 controls representing the general population. Although case-control studies do not establish causation, strong evidence in favor of an association between ER and VF-related SCD emerged.

Tikkanen and colleagues[4] systemically reported the long-term outcome of ER in the general population. The authors assessed the prevalence and prognostic significance of ER on routine ECG performed during a community-based investigational coronary artery disease study involving 10,864 middle-aged subjects. The mean follow-up was 30 ± 11 years with the primary end point of cardiac death and secondary end points of all-cause mortality and arrhythmic death. The prevalence of ER was 5.8% in this cohort. Importantly, ER in the inferior leads was found to be associated with an increased risk of cardiac death (adjusted relative risk [RR], 1.28; 95% confidence interval [CI], 1.04–1.59; P = .03) in the general population. J-point elevation in the lateral leads was of borderline significance in predicting cardiac death and all-cause death. Moreover, the survival curves started to diverge 15 years after the first ECG recording in the early 1980s and continued to diverge at a constant rate throughout the follow-up period, despite continued improvement in the treatment and prognosis of patients with cardiac disease during the past two decades. Although authors retrospectively classified cardiac deaths into arrhythmic and nonarrhythmic categories, the results strongly challenge the long-held benignancy of ER.

On the other hand, 59 out of 630 subjects with ER in the general population died of a proved arrhythmic cause over a mean period of 30 ± 11 years. Considering these data, the prevalence of so-called malignant ER turns out to be 1 per 10 cases with ER pattern on ECG, proving that 9 out of 10 cases with ER on ECG should really have been benign. In addition, the multivariate adjusted risk of all-cause mortality associated with presence of ER in any region and magnitude was not reported.

PATHOPHYSIOLOGY OF ER (MECHANISM)
Insights from Experimental Studies

The exact mechanism for ER is still unknown. In 1991, Antzelevitch and colleagues[28] first proposed that transmural differences in early phases of cardiac action potential (phases 1 and 2) are probably responsible for inscription of the ECG J wave. Subsequently, they obtained direct evidence in support of this hypothesis in arterially perfused canine ventricular wedge preparations in 1996.[29] Briefly, arrhythmogenic platform is created by disproportionate amplification of repolarizing current in the epicardial myocardium because of a decrease in inward sodium or calcium channel currents or an increase in outward potassium currents mediated by I_{to}, I_{K-ATP}, and I_{K-Ach} channels. The trigger and substrate for development of phase 2 reentry and VT/VF eventually emerge from the transmural dispersion in the duration of cardiac action potentials.

Insights from Genetic Testing

Because ER was only recently associated with increased risk of SCD, the genetic markers differentiating benign and arrhythmic forms of ER have not been identified. The importance of the genetic background in ER has recently been suggested by Haïssaguerre and colleagues[3] when they showed that 16% of cases with VF and ER have a family history of SCD.

Given the high frequency of the genetic background underlying the ER pattern in the population, it is probably polygenic and influenced by environmental factors. One could hypothesize that common variants contribute to the ECG pattern of ER and that a combination of such variants or the co-segregation of common and rare variants leads to the malignant form of ER. Large multicentric studies using state-of-the-art genomics approaches on large cohorts with malignant forms of ER patients should lead to the identification of the underlying molecular bases in this lethal arrhythmia.

As described previously, rare monogenic forms of ER have been reported using a candidate gene approach. ER on ECG suggests a shift in transmural voltage gradient between epicardium and endocardium as a causal mechanism. An increase in I_{to}, I_{Kr}, I_{Ks}, I_{KACH}, and I_{KATP} current or a decrease of sodium I_{Na} or calcium I_{CaL} current could lead to this phenomenon.

Following these hypotheses, a candidate gene approach on 156 probands allowed the identification of a rare variant in KCNJ8,[30] responsible for the pore-forming subunit of the I_{KATP} channel, in a 14-year-old girl who was resuscitated after an episode of sudden death caused by VF with ER syndrome. Her coronary angiogram with ergonovine injection, MRI, and flecainide and isoproterenol challenge tests were normal. She experienced more than 100 episodes of recurrent VF unresponsive to β-blockers, lidocaine-mexiletine, verapamil, and amiodarone. Recurrences of VF were associated with massive accentuation of the ER pattern at times mimicking acute myocardial ischemia. Coronary angiography during an episode with 1.2-mV J-ST elevation was normal. Isoproterenol infusion acutely suppressed electrical storms, whereas quinidine eliminated all recurrences of VF and restored a normal ECG, which has persisted over a follow-up of 65 months. The precise pathophysiologic mechanism is still being studied using in vitro reexpression of the mutant channel.

Burashnikov and colleagues[31] identified a missense variant in the β2 subunit of the cardiac L-type calcium channel in patients with ER syndrome. Expression studies for this variant are not yet available.

In parallel familial studies, several large pedigrees with malignant ER forms with autosomal-dominant pattern of inheritance have been identified. In each of these families the prevalence rates of SCD and ER are higher than in the general population. A strong genetic background has been suspected in a large pedigree of 66 members with 11 (16.6%) SCDs and two individuals with ER pattern (**Fig. 2**). Seven out of 11 SCDs occurred in individuals less than 35 years of age. Also, 11 (16.6%) asymptomatic individuals have an ER pattern. Furthermore, all the disease transmitters were identified to have variable expression of ER on ECG (slight notch at the end of the QRS). An ECG showing ER and VF before sudden death is

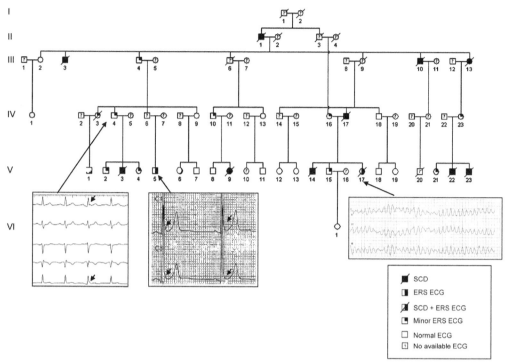

Fig. 2. Pedigree chart of 66 members with family history of electrocardiographic early repolarization syndrome (ERS ECG) and sudden cardiac death (SCD).

available only for patient V-17. In a second pedigree, individuals across three generations suffered SCD and five out of eight siblings have ER pattern (data not shown). Classical genetic linkage analysis assuming an autosomal-dominant form of inheritance of ER should allow identification of the disease-causing gene.

These data suggest an association between ER and SCD not only at a population level but also at a familial level demonstrating that ER ECG pattern could be considered as a malignant syndrome associated with a high risk of SCD in some families. The familial pattern undermines the need for systematic familial screening for the identification of ER to limit the risk of sudden death within the family.

Early Repolarization or Delayed Depolarization: a Controversy on the Origin of J Wave

Although the J wave is synonymously used with ER abnormality, the mechanistic evidence elucidating the inscription of J wave on surface ECG is incomplete. Basic investigators propose the inscription of J wave as coincident with phase 1 of cardiac action potential in the epicardial region of the ventricular myocardium, which precedes phase 1 in the endo- and mid-myocardial cells generating an early gradient in the repolarization currents within the

ventricles, thereby justifying J wave as an ER phenomenon.[28,29] In accordance with this, some clinical investigators concluded that J wave should be considered as a repolarization phenomenon rather than late depolarization because of its slower inscription, spontaneous and rate-dependant fluctuation in morphologic pattern (increased pattern at slow heart rate, decreased pattern at faster heart rate) or amplitude in the face of stable QRS complexes, and amplitude varying concurrently with ST segment. These investigators did not find late potentials on high-amplification electrocardiography and invasive endocardial mapping further reinforcing their view.[3]

In a recent work on deciphering the pathophysiology of J wave in ER syndrome,[32] 22 idiopathic VF patients were monitored for 24 hours using a newly developed signal-averaging system to record late potentials (depolarization marker); T-wave alternans; and QT dispersion (repolarization markers). Frequency-domain heart rate variability, which reflects autonomic modulation, also was assessed. The incidence of late potentials in 7 (32%) of 22 patients with VF and ER was higher than in the remaining 15 VF patients without ER (86% vs 27%; $P = .02$). In contrast, repolarization markers did not differ between the two groups. Moreover, dynamic changes in late potential parameters (fragmented QRS [fQRS], RMS_{40}, and LAS_{40}) were observed and were pronounced at nighttime only in the patients with VF and ER and high-frequency components (vagal tone index) on frequency-domain heart rate variability analysis were associated with J waves in VF patients ($P<.05$). These investigators concluded that because idiopathic VF patients with ER had a high incidence of late potentials showing circadian variation with night ascendancy, J waves caused by ER may be more closely associated with depolarization abnormality and autonomic modulation than with repolarization abnormality.

RELATIONSHIP BETWEEN J WAVE ELEVATION AND VF
Amplitude of J Wave

Amplitude of J wave is more important in VF patients compared with controls (2.15 ± 1.2 mm in IVF vs 1.05 ± 0.2 mm).[3] Tikkanen and colleagues[4] reported higher relative risk of cardiac death with a J point elevation of 0.2 mV (RR 3.03; 95% CI, 1.88–4.90; $P = .001$) compared with 0.1 mV (RR 1.30; 95% CI, 1.05–1.61; $P = .02$).

Spontaneous Dynamicity

Because most of the VF episodes cannot be predicted clinically in patients with sporadic episodes of VF, it is difficult to gain further insight into the role of ER in the mechanism of VF. However, some of the patients with VF experience electrical storm during hospitalization, unraveling the dynamics of ER in VF arrhythmogenesis. Haïssaguerre and colleagues[33] performed serial ECGs during electrical storm (including frequent ventricular ectopy and episodes of VF) in 16 subjects and all patients showed consistent and marked increase in the amplitude of J wave during the period of storm when compared with baseline pattern (from 2.6 ± 1 mm to 4.1 ± 2 mm; $P<.001$). Besides spontaneous accentuation of the J-wave amplitude preceding electrical storm, spontaneous beat-to-beat fluctuation in the morphologic pattern of ER was also observed.[3] Out of 11 patients with VF and ER reported by Nam and colleagues,[11] 5 patients experienced VF storm during their stay in intensive care unit. ECGs recorded within 30 minutes of the VF storm exhibited global appearance of J waves. These dynamic ECG features of ER appeared spontaneously for a transient period around the VF storm revealing the presence of a functional "substrate" for arrhythmia.

Correlation Between J Point Location and Arrhythmia Origin

The authors mapped patients with ER and VF targeting the ventricular ectopy initiating the VF. In patients with ER recorded in inferior leads alone, all ectopies originated from the inferior left ventricular wall. In the subjects with widespread global ER, as recorded in both inferior and lateral leads, ectopy originated from multiple regions.[3,34] These findings prove that ER abnormality may be either limited to a single region in the ventricles or can extend beyond it to involve more than one region simultaneously. Whether or not J wave truly represents an abnormality of repolarization is still debated,[35] but these findings help toward localizing ER as an abnormality involving distal Purkinje tissue, its innervated myocardium, or the Purkinje-myocardial junctions.

RISK STRATIFICATION

As described previously, although ER is a common entity, unexplained sudden cardiac arrest in young adults is very rare. Some investigators addressed this issue by using the Bayes' law of conditional probabilities. Rosso and colleagues[10] claimed that the presence of J wave in a young adult would increase the probability of VF from 3.4:100,000 to 11:100,000, which is a negligible rise. They concluded that the incidental discovery of J wave on routine screening should not be interpreted as a marker of "high risk" for sudden death because the odds for this fatal disease would still be approximately 1:10,000. Now the question is: "how to differentiate subjects with 'high risk' ER from the so-called benign ER?"

Clinical Features

In such a situation, we consider that close follow-up should be offered to patients with ER and unexplained syncope or a family history of unexplained sudden death. Abe and colleagues[36] reported that the prevalence of ER in 222 patients with syncope and no organic disorder was 18.5%, which is almost 10 times that in 3915 healthy controls (2%). Therefore, the possibility of ER-associated syncopal episodes cannot be excluded in at least some of these patients. The genetic basis of ER is still largely unknown. Also, in patients with VF and ER, positive family history of sudden death was not significantly higher than in those without ER (16% vs 9%; $P = .17$).[3] Nevertheless, it does not imply that family history is not an important aspect of history-taking in ER patients.

Magnitude of J Wave

In the study by Tikkanen and colleagues,[4] subjects with J-point elevation of more than 0.2 mV on inferior leads not only bore a higher risk of death from cardiac causes (adjusted RR, 2.98; 95% CI,

1.85–4.92; P<.001) as compared with J-point elevation of more than 0.1 mV, but also had a markedly elevated risk of death from arrhythmia (adjusted RR, 2.92; 95% CI, 1.45–5.89; P = .01). This finding indicates that the magnitude of J-point elevation could be a discriminator of risk. However, this study did not provide the sensitivity and specificity of this measure in predicting the end point events. In accordance with this finding, Haïssaguerre and colleagues[3] also found that the magnitude of J-wave elevation in case group was significantly higher than that in control subjects (2 ± 0.8 mV vs 1.2 ± 0.4 mV; P<.001). It is noteworthy that J-point elevation of more than 0.2 mV seems rare in the normal population. In 630 of 10,864 subjects with ER identified by Tikkanen and colleagues,[4] 0.33% of the total population had J-wave elevation of more than 0.2 mV. However, it is also necessary to point out that the magnitude of J-wave elevation can fluctuate even without drug provocation or exercise. This means that low magnitude of J wave should not be considered as a static entity. It can potentially get augmented. Unfortunately, currently there is no reliable provocation test to augment ER in inferolateral leads.

Distribution of J Waves

In normal subjects, most of the ER is confined to inferior leads, lateral leads (I/aVL) or left precordial leads. As reported by Tikkanen and colleagues,[4] out of 630 subjects with ER, only 16 subjects (2.5%) had ER in both the inferior and lateral leads. Focusing on patients with VF, Haïssaguerre and colleagues[3] found that 46.9% of patients with VF and ER had ER in both inferior and lateral leads. Similarly, global presence of ER was observed in

none of the 46 subjects with ER without VF (selected from among 1395 individuals from the general population) but in 45.5% of patients with ER who developed VF.[11]

Morphology of J Waves

Recently, Merchant and colleagues[37] compared the baseline ECGs between nine patients with VF/VT and ER (so-called "malignant ER" group) and 61 age- and gender-matched controls with normal ER (so-called "benign ER" group). The results demonstrated that QRS notching was more prevalent among cases than controls in leads V4 (44% vs 5%; P = .001); V5 (44% vs 8%; P = .006); and V6 (33% vs 5%; P = .013). They concluded that left precordial terminal QRS notching is more prevalent in malignant variants of ER than in benign cases and could be used as a tool for risk stratification of subjects with ER. However, the case number in this study is small and it includes three patients with idiopathic monomorphic VT without VF.

Fragmented QRS

Liu and colleagues[38] looked at –fQRS (defined as presence of ≥1 additional deflections or notching within the QRS complex including top of R wave or nadir of S wave) in at least two contiguous leads of 16 ICD recipients with VF and ER. Seven patients (43.8%) had fQRS in two to four (mean: 2.7) leads and after a mean follow-up of 67 ± 66 months, five (71.4%) of seven patients had recurrent VF (ICD shocks ranging from one to eight, mean 3.8) (Fig. 3). None of the nine patients lacking fQRS experienced appropriate ICD discharges (P<.01). The authors concluded that the presence of fQRS, indicating depolarization disturbance,

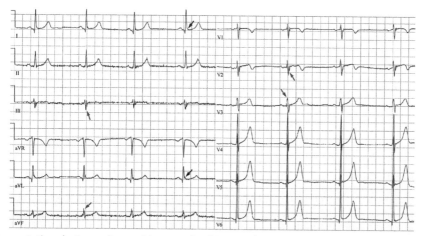

Fig. 3. A representative electrocardiographic example of J wave elevation in lateral leads (*black arrows*) and fragmentation of the QRS (*red arrows*) associated with recurrent ventricular fibrillation.

increases the risk of recurrent ventricular arrhythmias in patients with VF and ER.

Invasive Induction of VF

Induction of VF was attempted in 132 VF patients from two different ventricular sites and up to three extrastimuli with shortest coupling interval of 209 ± 30 ms. The patients with ER did not show significantly higher inducibility than those without ER (16 of 47 vs 17 of 85; $P = .07$).[3] Moreover, a low rate of VF inducibility (34%) in the patients with ER Syndrome (VF + ECG pattern) makes electrophysiologic study less sensitive in risk stratification of asymptomatic patients.

MANAGEMENT OF VF ASSOCIATED WITH ER

Patients with VF and ER have shown higher incidence of VF recurrence than VF patients without ER (43% vs 23%; $P<0.001$) during 5 years of follow-up. Moreover, out of 122 patients with VF and ER, 33 (27%) patients experienced more than three episodes of VF and 16 experienced electrical storm (≥3 VF per 24 hours). Based on these observations, the patients with VF and ER may be the candidates for treatment over and above an implantable defibrillator. In this population, acute control of arrhythmia could be achieved by deep sedation or isoproterenol infusion. Quinidine was effective in preventing the recurrence during follow-up. Interestingly, ER pattern was closely linked to the period of occurrence of arrhythmia and was helpful to monitor the efficacy of drug therapy. At the time of arrhythmia occurrence, ER was more pronounced than during the period without arrhythmia (**Fig. 4**). Amiodarone, β-blockers, and Class IC drugs were ineffective in establishing control of recurrent VF.[33]

Catheter ablation of the ectopy initiating the VF could be another potential modality in the management of VF patients with ER who fail to respond to drugs. In a small number of patients who underwent invasive mapping of the ectopy, six out of eight subjects with ER in the inferior leads, ectopy originated from the inferior left ventricular wall. In the remaining two patients with inferolateral ER, ectopy originated from multiple regions. Catheter ablation eliminated all ectopies in five subjects.[3]

J-WAVE SYNDROMES

Other conditions that display J-wave elevation include acquired (myocardial ischemia, hypothermia, hypercalcemia, and so forth) and inherited (Brugada syndrome) disorders. As for variants of long QT syndrome, different types of J-wave elevation are responsible for malignant ventricular arrhythmia caused by different molecular or regional abnormalities. ER has been reported to be present in 12% of Brugada syndrome patients. The significance of this association is unclear.

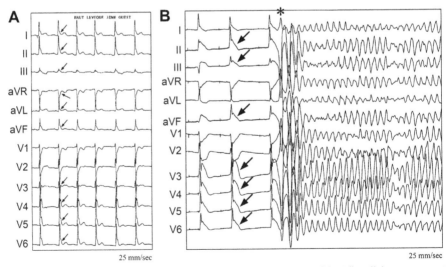

Fig. 4. (*A*) Baseline ECG of a survivor of sudden cardiac arrest (16-year-old girl). All known structural heart diseases and primary electrical diseases, including long/short QT syndrome, Brugada syndrome, and catecholamine-sensitive ventricular tachycardia were excluded in this patient. The only significant finding on the ECG was a prominent J wave (*arrows*) as can be seen in almost all the leads other than V1 and V2. (*B*) During the electrophysiologic study, an episode of spontaneous ventricular fibrillation (VF) was triggered by a ventricular ectopy with very short coupling interval (*asterisk*). Note the J wave in the inferior and precordial leads (*arrows*) gets significantly augmented before the occurrence VF than at the baseline. Sweep speed, 25 mm/s.

Table 2
Similarities and differences between early repolarization syndrome and Brugada syndrome

Characteristics	Early Repolarization Syndrome	Brugada Syndrome
Similarities		
Gender preponderance	Male	Male
Age at diagnosis	Around 40 y	Around 40 y
Situation favoring arrhythmia	Rest/sleep	Rest/sleep
Effective therapy of recurrent VF	Isoproterenol/quinidine	Isoproterenol/quinidine
Autonomic influence	Vagal tone	Vagal tone
Differences		
ECG localization	II, III, aVF; V5, V6; I, aVL	V1–V3
ST pattern	Slur/notch	Coved type
Conduction	Normal	Often abnormal
Sodium channel blocker effect	None	Accentuation
VF sources	Left ventricle ± right ventricle	Right ventricle
Genetic mutations	None	SCN5A, GPD1-L, CACNA1C, CACNB2B

Two studies that looked at the outcome in these patients reported mutually conflicting results (no difference vs increased risk).[39,40]

Even if some similarities exist between the ER and the Brugada syndrome, some major differences favor ER syndrome as a distinct entity (**Table 2**). First, both ECG patterns were considered as normal variant before the 1990s.[14,41] Second, similar mechanism was experimentally demonstrated by Yan and Antzelevitch[29] to explain J-wave elevation in both syndromes. Both syndromes are associated with ventricular arrhythmias at rest (± vagal period) predominantly in young men in their late 30s or early 40s. Finally, recurrent VF associated with these syndromes responds similarly to isoproterenol acutely and quinidine as a long-term secondary prevention therapy.[42,43] Regarding the differences between the two syndromes, Brugada syndrome differs from the ER syndrome in terms of regional ECG location (V1–V3 vs inferolateral leads) and morphology of J-point elevation (coved-type vs slurring or notching). No conduction disorders were found in any patients with VF and ER pattern, whereas they have been commonly found in Brugada syndrome. Sodium channel blockers provoke or accentuate the ECG pattern in Brugada syndrome; it does not alter or attenuate (ajmaline) the ER pattern. To conclude, a mutation in SCN5A has been found in 20% of patients with Brugada syndrome but in none of the 135 patients with ER syndrome and VF who have been genotyped. Only sporadic variants of KCNJ8, CACNA1C, and CACNB2B have been reported in patients with ER and VF.[30,31]

SUMMARY

Current scientific evidence drawn from a large cohort of subjects with long-term follow-up suggests that J-wave elevation in the inferolateral leads is not always benign. There is a high prevalence of ER in patients experiencing first, recurrent, and stormy episodes of idiopathic VF. Careful evaluation of patients having ER associated with unexplained syncope, family history of SCD, or idiopathic ventricular arrhythmias is recommended. It is particularly important to pay attention in the case of J wave greater than 0.2 mV, global J wave, and notched J wave in the left precordial leads.

REFERENCES

1. Zipes DP, Wellens HJJ. Sudden cardiac death. Circulation 1998;98:2334–51.
2. Huikuri HV, Castellanos A, Myerburg RJ. Sudden death due to cardiac arrhythmias. N Engl J Med 2001;345:1473–82.
3. Haïssaguerre M, Derval N, Sacher F, et al. Sudden cardiac arrest associated with early repolarization. N Engl J Med 2008;358:2016–23.
4. Tikkanen JT, Anttonen O, Junttila MJ, et al. Long-term outcome associated with early repolarization on electrocardiography. N Engl J Med 2009;361:2529–37.

5. Klatsky AL, Oehm R, Cooper RA, et al. The early repolarization normal variant electrocardiogram: correlates and consequences. Am J Med 2003;115:171–7.

6. Mehta M, Jain AC, Mehta A. Early repolarization. Clin Cardiol 1999;22:59–65.

7. Tomaszewski W. Changement electrocardiographiques observes chez un homme mort de froid. Arch Mal Coeur Vaiss 1938;31:525–8.

8. Osborn JJ. Experimental hypothermia: respiratory and blood pH changes in relation to cardiac function. Am J Physiol 1953;175:389–98.

9. Marcus RR, Kalisetti D, Raxwal V, et al. Early repolarization in patients with spinal cord injury: prevalence and clinical significance. J Spinal Cord Med 2002; 25:33–8.

10. Rosso R, Kogan E, Belhassen B, et al. J-point elevation in survivors of primary ventricular fibrillation and matched control subjects: incidence and clinical significance. J Am Coll Cardiol 2008;52:1231–48.

11. Nam GB, Ko KH, Kim J, et al. Mode of onset of ventricular fibrillation in patients with early repolarization pattern vs Brugada syndrome. Eur Heart J 2010;31(3):330–9.

12. Kui C, Congxin H, Xi W, et al. Characteristic of the prevalence of J wave in apparently healthy Chinese adults. Arch Med Res 2008;39:232–45.

13. Nam GB, Kim YH, Antzelevitch C. Augmentation of J waves and electrical storms in patients with early repolarization. N Engl J Med 2008;358:2078–209.

14. Goldman MJ. RS-T segment elevation in mid- and left precordial leads as a normal variant. Am Heart J 1953;46:817–20.

15. Grusin H. Peculiarities of the African's electrocardiogram and the changes observed in serial studies. Circulation 1954;9:860–87.

16. Goldman MJ. Normal variants in the electrocardiogram leading to cardiac invalidism. Am Heart J 1960;59:71–7.

17. Wasserburger RH. The normal RS-T segment elevation variant. Am J Cardiol 1961;8:184–92.

18. Fenichel NN. A long term study of concave RS-T elevation: a normal variant of the electrocardiogram. Angiology 1962;13:360–6.

19. Kambara H, Phillips J. Long-term evaluation of early repolarization syndrome (normal variant RS-T segment elevation). Am J Cardiol 1976;38:157–61.

20. Kalla H, Yan GX, Marinchak R. Ventricular fibrillation in a patient with prominent J (Osborn) waves and ST segment elevation in the inferior electrocardiographic leads: a Brugada syndrome variant? J Cardiovasc Electrophysiol 2000;11:95–8.

21. Tsunoda Y, Taketshi Y, Nozaki N, et al. Presence of intermittent J waves in multiple leads in relation to episode of atrial and ventricular fibrillation. J Electrocardiol 2004;37:311–34.

22. Ogawa M, Kumagai K, Yamanouchi Y, et al. Spontaneous onset of ventricular fibrillation in Brugada syndrome with J wave and ST-segment elevation in the inferior leads. Heart Rhythm 2005;2:97–9.

23. Gussak I, Antzelevitch C. Early repolarization syndrome: clinical characteristics and possible cellular and ionic mechanisms. J Electrocardiol 2000;33:299–309.

24. Yan GX, Yao QH, Wang DQ, et al. Electrocardiographic J wave and J wave syndromes. Chin J Cardiac Arrhyth 2004;8:360–5.

25. Shu J, Zhu T, Yang L, et al. ST-segment elevation in the early repolarization syndrome, idiopathic ventricular fibrillation, and the Brugada syndrome: cellular and clinical linkage. J Electrocardiol 2005;38:26–32.

26. Hlaing T, Dimino T, Kowey PR, et al. ECG repolarization waves: their genesis and clinical implications. Ann Noninvasive Electrocardiol 2005;10:211–23.

27. Haïssaguerre M, Sacher F, Derval N, et al. Early repolarization in the inferolateral leads: a new syndrome associated with sudden cardiac death. J Interv Card Electrophysiol 2007;18:281.

28. Antzelevitch C, Sicouri S, Litovsky SH, et al. Heterogeneity within the ventricular wall. Electrophysiology and pharmacology of epicardial, endocardial, and M cells. Circ Res 1991;69:1427–49.

29. Yan GX, Antzelevitch C. Cellular basis for the electrocardiographic J wave. Circulation 1996;93: 372–9.

30. Haïssaguerre M, Chatel S, Sacher F, et al. Ventricular fibrillation with prominent early repolarization associated with a rare variant of KCNJ8/KATP channel. J Cardiovasc Electrophysiol 2009;20(1):93–8.

31. Burashnikov E, Pfeifer R, Borgreffe M, et al. Mutations in the cardiac L-type calcium channel associated with inherited sudden cardiac death syndromes. Circulation 2009;120:S573 [abstract].

32. Abe A, Ikeda T, Tsukada T, et al. Circadian variation of late potentials in idiopathic ventricular fibrillation associated with J waves: insights into alternative pathophysiology and risk stratification. Heart Rhythm 2010;7(5):675–82.

33. Haissaguerre M, Sacher F, Nogami A, et al. Characteristics of recurrent ventricular fibrillation associated with inferolateral early repolarization role of drug therapy. J Am Coll Cardiol 2009;53:612–9.

34. Sacher F, Derval N, Jesel L, et al. Initiation of ventricular arrhythmia in idiopathic ventricular fibrillation associated with early repolarization syndrome. Heart Rhythm 2008;5S:S150, PO1–136.

35. Borggrefe M, Schimpf R. J-wave syndromes caused by repolarization or depolarization mechanisms a debated issue among experimental and clinical electrophysiologists. J Am Coll Cardiol 2010;55(8): 798–800.

36. Abe A, Yoshino H, Ishiguro H, et al. Prevalence of J waves in 12-lead electrocardiogram in patients with syncope and no organic disorder. J Cardiovasc Electrophysiol 2007;18(Suppl 2):S88.

37. Merchant FM, Noseworthy PA, Weiner RB, et al. Ability of terminal QRS notching to distinguish benign from malignant electrocardiographic forms of early repolarization. Am J Cardiol 2009;104:1402–6.

38. Liu X, Hocini M, Derval N, et al. Fragmented QRS complexes as a predictor of ventricular arrhythmic events in patients with idiopathic ventricular fibrillation and early repolarization [abstract]. Heart Rhythm 2010;7(5):S175.

39. Letsas KP, Sacher F, Probst V, et al. Prevalence of early repolarization pattern in inferolateral leads in patients with Brugada syndrome. Heart Rhythm 2008;5(12):1685–9.

40. Sarkozy A, Chierchia GB, Paparella G, et al. Inferior and lateral electrocardiographic repolarization abnormalities in Brugada syndrome. Circ Arrhythm Electrophysiol 2009;2(2):154–61.

41. Edeiken J. Elevation of the RS-T segment, apparent or real, in the right precordial leads as a probable normal variant. Am Heart J 1954;48(3):331–9.

42. Belhassen B, Glick A, Viskin S. Efficacy of quinidine in high-risk patients with Brugada syndrome. Circulation 2004;110(13):1731–7.

43. Hermida JS, Denjoy I, Clerc J, et al. Hydroquinidine therapy in Brugada syndrome. J Am Coll Cardiol 2004;43(10):1853–60.

Arrhythmogenic Right Ventricular Cardiomyopathy

Koji Fukuzawa, MD, PhD[a], Alessandro Zorzi, MD[a],
Federico Migliore, MD[a], Ilaria Rigato, MD, PhD[a],
Barbara Bauce, MD, PhD[a], Cristina Basso, MD, PhD[b],
Gaetano Thiene, MD[b], Domenico Corrado, MD, PhD[a],*

KEYWORDS

- Arrhythmogenic right ventricular cardiomyopathy
- Sudden cardiac death • Ventricular arrhythmia • Genetics
- Catheter ablation • Implantable cardioverter defibrillator

Arrhythmogenic right ventricular cardiomyopathy (ARVC) is an inheritable heart muscle disease characterized by fibrofatty replacement of the right ventricular (RV) myocardium.[1–6] Clinical manifestations are related to electrical instability, including either ventricular tachycardia (VT) of RV origin or ventricular fibrillation (VF), which may lead to sudden death, mostly in young people or athletes. Ventricular arrhythmias get worse during or immediately after exercise and participation in competitive athletics has been associated with an increased risk for sudden death.[7,8] Later in the disease history, the RV becomes more diffusely involved and left ventricular (LV) involvement may result in biventricular heart failure.[5,6]

The estimated prevalence of ARVC in the general population ranges from 1 in 2000 to 1 in 5000. A familial background has been demonstrated in about 50% of ARVC cases. The disease affects men more frequently than women (with a ratio up to 3:1) and becomes clinically overt most often in the third or fourth decade of life.[4,9–11]

Clinical diagnosis of ARVC is often difficult because of the nonspecific nature of the disease and the broad spectrum of phenotypic manifestation, ranging from severe to concealed forms. In 1994[12] and 2010,[13] The International Task Force proposed criteria for the clinical diagnosis of ARVC.

ARVC shows an autosomal dominant pattern of inheritance with incomplete penetrance and variable clinical expression,[14] although an autosomal recessive variant has been identified.[15,16] Since the first ARVC-causing gene (ie, plakoglobin gene- JUP) was identified in patients with Naxos disease, several mutations of genes encoding desmosomal cell adhesion proteins have been detected in patients with ARVC.[9–11] Molecular genetic analysis is a powerful tool for preclinical diagnosis of ARVC in asymptomatic family members of gene-positive probands and may contribute to risk stratification and clinical management.

The most important therapeutic objective in ARVC is to prevent arrhythmic sudden death. The implantable cardioverter defibrillator (ICD) is the most effective tool against arrhythmic sudden death although antiarrhythmic drugs (AADs) and catheter ablation may play a role for treatment of nonlife-threatening arrhythmia.

This review article addresses the clinical presentation, the diagnosis, and the advancements on molecular biology of ARVC, and how these advancements have impacted on understanding

Disclosures: No other potential conflict of interest relevant to this article was reported.
[a] Department of Cardiac Thoracic and Vascular Sciences, University of Padua Medical School, University of Padua, Via Giustiniani 2, 35121, Padova, Italy
[b] Department of Medico-Diagnostic Sciences and Special Therapies, University of Padua Medical School, University of Padua, Via Gabelli 61, 35121, Italy
* Corresponding author.
E-mail address: domenico.corrado@unipd.it

disease pathogenesis, diagnosis, and establishing management strategies.

CLINICAL PRESENTATION
Symptoms and Family History

Palpitation or syncope caused by isolated premature ventricular beats or VT of RV origin is the most common clinical presentation, and these clinical symptoms become clinically overt most often in the third or fourth decade of life.[4,9-11] However, sudden cardiac death sometimes occurs as the first clinical presentation in young individuals. Later in disease history, symptoms caused by RV or biventricular failure become apparent in some patients with ARVC.[5,6]

Familial background has been identified in 50% of patients with ARVC. Once a proband is diagnosed with the disease, cascade screening is indicated for the detection of affected family members before their clinical symptoms become evident.

Morphologic Abnormalities

The spectrum of RV alterations ranges from global RV dilatation/dysfunction to regional wall motion abnormalities or bulges typically localized in the triangle of dysplasia, (ie, subtricuspid, apical, and infundibular regions [**Fig. 1**]).[2,5,6] The LV and the septum are usually involved to a lesser extent; whereas, biventricular or left dominant variants of disease have been reported.[4-6]

Depolarization/Repolarization Abnormalities

Electrocardiogram (ECG) depolarization abnormalities are caused by a right intraventricular conduction defect. They include prolongation of

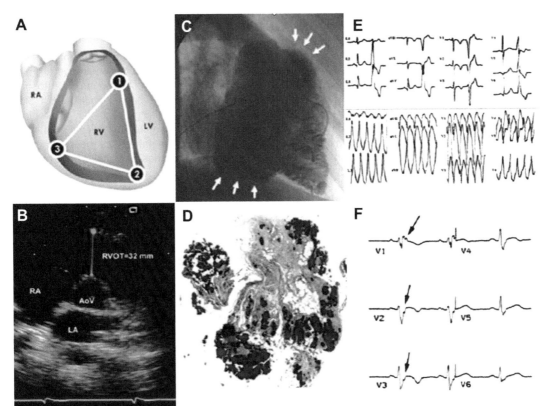

Fig. 1. Morpho-functional, electrocardiographic, and tissue characterization diagnostic features of ARVC. (A) Diagram of the triangle of dysplasia, which illustrates the characteristic areas for structural and functional abnormalities of the RV. (B) Two-dimensional echocardiography showing RV outflow tract enlargement from the parasternal short-axis view. (C) Right ventricular contrast angiography (30° right anterior-oblique view) demonstrating a localized RV outflow tract aneurysm (arrows) as well as infero-basal akinesia (arrows) with mild tricuspid regurgitation. (D) Endomyocardial biopsy sample with extensive myocardial atrophy and fibrofatty replacement (trichrome; x6). (E) 12-lead ECG with inverted T waves (V₁, V₂, V₃), with LBBB morphology premature ventricular beats and VT. (F) ECG tracing showing postexcitation epsilon wave in precordial leads V_1, V_2, V_3 (arrows). AoV, aortic valve; LA, left atrium; LV, left ventricle; RA, right atrium; RV, right ventricle; RVOT, right ventricle outflow tract. (Modified from Basso C, Corrado D, Marcus FI, et al. Arrhythmogenic right ventricular cardiomyopathy. Lancet 2009;373:1289-30; with permission.)

QRS interval (≥110 milliseconds) or epsilon waves in right precordial leads,[17-19] incomplete/complete right bundle branch block, and late potentials by signal average ECG (see **Fig. 1**).[20]

T-wave inversion in the right precordial leads (V1−V2/V3) is the most common repolarization abnormality. QT/QRS dispersion across 12-leads ECG was reported to be a noninvasive predictor of an increased risk of sudden cardiac death.[21]

Ventricular Arrhythmia

Ventricular arrhythmia usually shows a left bundle branch block morphology, which suggests RV origin (see **Fig. 1**). The severity of arrhythmia ranges from isolated premature ventricular beats to sustained VT and VF.[4-6] VF often occurs in young individuals and competitive athletes as the first clinical sign of the disease. Instead, macro-reentrant monomorphic VT, which is associated with myocardial scar, is more common in a later phase of disease.[14]

DIAGNOSIS
Original and Modified Task Force Criteria

The 1994 Task Force Criteria were initially designed to guarantee an adequate specificity for ARVC among index cases with overt clinical manifestations.[12] However, The 1994 Criteria lack sensitivity for identification of early/minor phenotypes, particularly in the setting of familial ARVC. Accordingly, diagnostic criteria have been recently revised with the aim of improving diagnostic sensitivity.[13] Comparison of original versus revised criteria is presented in **Table 1**. The approach of classifying structural, histopathologic, ECG, arrhythmic, and genetic features of the disease as major and minor criteria has been maintained. As far as ECG and arrhythmic features, in the revised Task Force Criteria T-wave inversion in V1 to V3 as well as VT with left bundle branch block (LBBB) morphology with superior/indeterminate QRS axis, either sustained or nonsustained, have become major criteria. The following findings have been included among minor criteria: (1) T-wave inversion in V1 and V2 in the absence of right bundle branch block (RBBB), and from V1 to V4 in the presence of complete RBBB; (2) positivity of any one of the 3 signal-averaged ECG (SAECG) parameters for late potentials; and (3) premature ventricular beats greater than 500 per 24 hours on the Holter monitoring. Moreover, revised guidelines provide quantitative cutoff values in imaging and histopathological criteria. Finally, the identification of a pathogenetic gene mutation in a first-degree relative has become a major criterion for ARVC diagnosis.

CLINICAL IMPACT OF MOLECULAR GENETICS
Genetic Background

The inherited nature of ARVC has been recognized since 1982 when Marcus and colleagues[22] described 24 adult cases, 2 of those were from the same family. In 1988, a report on 9 Italian families, demonstrated for the first time the autosomal dominant pattern of inheritance with incomplete penetrance and variable expression.[23]

The first ARVC-causing gene (ie, the plakoglobin gene [JUP]), was identified in patients with Naxos disease, a syndrome characterized by palmoplantar keratosis, woolly hair, and ARVC with an autosomal recessive pattern of inheritance.[15] Plakoglobin protein is a component of desmosomes, which are specialized intercellular structures providing mechanical attachment of myocytes. A schematic representation of desmosomal complex is depicted in **Fig. 2** and the summary of ARVC-causing genes are shown in **Table 2**.

A cardio-cutaneous syndrome, similar to Naxos disease, mainly involving the LV has also been reported (so-called Carvajal disease). The cause of Carvajal syndrome is a defective desmoplakin gene (DSP).[16] Dominant forms of ARVC caused by DSP gene mutations were also identified.[24] A variety of mutations in plakophilin-2 (PKP-2) have been reported in almost one-third of unrelated probands from 3 different cohorts of subjects with ARVC across the world.[25-27] Subsequently, desmoglein-2 (DSG2)[28,29] and desmocollin-2 (DSC2)[30,31] were detected as rare disease-causing desmosomal genes.[32]

Other genes mutation unrelated to cell adhesion complex were also identified. Mutations in gene encoding cardiac ryanodine receptor (RyR2), which is responsible for calcium release from the sarcoplasmic reticulum and homeostasis, have been identified in an autosomal dominant form of ARVC.[33] Mutation of the TGFβ-3 gene was identified in clinically affected members of an ARVC family.[34] TGFβ3 can induce myocardial fibrosis and modulate expression of genes encoding desmosomal proteins in different cell types. Most recently, TMEM43 has been discovered as an ARVC-gene that causes a highly lethal and fully penetrant disease variant (ARVD5).[35] Little is known about the function of the TMEM43 gene, which may be a part of an adipogenic pathway regulated by PPARg, explaining the pathogenesis of fibrofatty replacement of the myocardium in ARVC.

Pathogenesis

The incorporation of defective proteins into cardiac desmosomes may provoke detachment of

Table 1
Comparison of Original and Revised Task Force Criteria

Original Task Force Criteria	Revised Task Force Criteria
I. Global or regional dysfunction and structural alterations[a]	
Major	**Major**
Severe dilatation and reduction of RV ejection fraction with no (or only mild) LV impairment	*By 2D echo*
Localized RV aneurysms (akinetic or dyskinetic areas with diastolic bulging)	Regional RV akinesia, dyskinesia, or aneurysm and 1 of the following (end diastole):
Severe segmental dilatation of the RV	PLAX RVOT ≥32 mm (corrected for body size [PLAX/BSA] ≥ 19 mm/m2)
	PSAX RVOT ≥36 mm (corrected for body size [PSAX/BSA] ≥21 mm/m2)
	or fractional area change ≤33%
	By MRI
	Regional RV akinesia or dyskinesia or dyssynchronous RV contraction and 1 of the following:
	Ratio of RV end-diastolic volume to BSA ≥110 mL/m2 (male) or ≥100 mL/m2 (female)
	or RV ejection fraction ≤40%
	By RV angiography
	Regional RV akinesia, dyskinesia, or aneurysm
Minor	**Minor**
Mild global RV dilatation or ejection fraction reduction with normal LV	*By 2D echo*
Mild segmental dilatation of the RV	Regional RV akinesia or dyskinesia and 1 of the following (end diastole):
Regional RV hypokinesia	PLAX RVOT ≥29 to <32 mm (corrected for body size [PLAX/BSA] ≥16 to <19 m/m2)
	PSAX RVOT ≥32 to <36 mm (corrected for body size [PSAX/BSA] ≥18 to <21 mm/m2)
	or fractional area change >33% to ≤40%
	By MRI
	Regional RV akinesia or dyskinesia or dyssynchronous RV contraction and 1 of the following:
	Ratio of RV end-diastolic volume to BSA ≥100 to <110 mL/m2 (male) or ≥90 to <100 mL/m2 (female)
	or RV ejection fraction >40% to ≤45%

II. Tissue characterization of wall

Major	Fibrofatty replacement of myocardium on endomyocardial biopsy	Residual myocytes <60% by morphometric analysis (or <50% if estimated), with fibrous replacement of the RV free wall myocardium in ≥1 sample, with or without fatty replacement of tissue on endomyocardial biopsy
Minor		Residual myocytes 60%–75% by morphometric analysis (or 50%–65% if estimated), with fibrous replacement of the RV free wall myocardium in ≥1 sample, with or without fatty replacement of tissue on endomyocardial biopsy

III. Repolarization abnormalities

Major	Inverted T waves in right precordial leads (V2 and V3) (people aged >12 years, in absence of right bundle-branch block)	Inverted T waves in right precordial leads (V1, V2, and V3) or beyond in individuals aged >14 years (in the absence of complete right bundle-branch block QRS ≥120 ms)
Minor	Inverted T waves in right precordial leads (V2 and V3) (people aged >12 years, in absence of right bundle-branch block)	Inverted T waves in leads V1 and V2 in individuals >14 years of age (in the absence of complete right bundle-branch block) or in V4, V5, or V6 Inverted T waves in leads V1, V2, V3, and V4 in individuals aged >14 years in the presence of complete right bundle-branch block

V. Depolarization/conduction abnormalities

Major	Epsilon waves or localized prolongation (>110 ms) of the QRS complex in right precordial leads (V1 to V3)	Epsilon wave (reproducible low-amplitude signals between end of QRS complex to onset of the T wave) in the right precordial leads (V1 to V3)
Minor	Late potentials (SAECG)	Late potentials by SAECG in ≥1 of 3 parameters in the absence of a QRS duration of ≥110 ms on the standard ECG Filtered QRS duration ≥114 ms Duration of terminal QRS <40 μV (low-amplitude signal duration) ≥38 ms Root-mean-square voltage of terminal 40 ms ≤20 μV Terminal activation duration of QRS ≥55 ms measured from the nadir of the S wave to the end of the QRS, including R in V1, V2, or V3, in the absence of complete right bundle-branch block

V. Arrhythmias

Major		Nonsustained or sustained ventricular tachycardia of left bundle-branch morphology with superior axis (negative or indeterminate QRS in leads II, III, and aVF and positive in lead aVL)

(continued on next page)

Table 1
(continued)

Original Task Force Criteria	Revised Task Force Criteria
Minor Left bundle-branch block–type ventricular tachycardia (sustained and nonsustained) (ECG, Holter, exercise) Frequent ventricular extrasystoles (>1000/24 h) (Holter)	Minor Nonsustained or sustained ventricular tachycardia of RV outflow configuration, left bundle-branch block morphology with inferior axis (positive QRS in leads II, III, and aVF and negative in lead aVL) or of unknown axis >500 ventricular extrasystoles per 24 h (Holter)
VI. Family history	
Major Familial disease confirmed at necropsy or surgery	Major ARVC confirmed in a first-degree relative who meets current Task Force Criteria ARVC confirmed pathologically at autopsy or surgery in a first-degree relative Identification of a pathogenic mutation[b] categorized as associated or probably associated with ARVC in the patient under evaluation.
Minor Family history of premature sudden death (<35 years of age) due to suspected ARVC familial history (clinical diagnosis based on present criteria)	Minor History of ARVC in a first-degree relative in whom it is not possible or practical to determine whether the family member meets current Task Force Criteria Premature sudden death (<35 years of age) due to suspected ARVC in a first-degree relative ARVC confirmed pathologically or by current Task Force Criteria in second-degree relative

Diagnostic terminology for original criteria: This diagnosis is fulfilled by the presence of 2 major criteria, 1 major plus 2 minor, or 4 minor criteria from different groups. Diagnostic terminology for revised criteria: definite diagnosis indicates 2 major or 1 major and 2 minor criteria or 4 minor from different categories; borderline indicates 1 major and 1 minor or 3 minor criteria from different categories; and possible indicates 1 major or 2 minor criteria from different categories.

Abbreviations: BSA, body surface area; PLAX, parasternal long-axis view; PSAX, parasternal short-axis view; SAECG, signal-averaged ECG.

[a] Hypokinesis is not included in this or subsequent definitions of RV regional wall motion abnormalities for the proposed modified criteria.

[b] A pathogenic mutation is a DNA alteration associated with that alters or is expected to alter the encoded protein, is unobserved, or rare in a large non-ARVC control population, and either alters or is predicted to alter the structure or function of the protein or has demonstrated linkage to the disease phenotype in a conclusive pedigree.

Modified from Marcus FI, McKenna WJ, Sherrill D, et al. Diagnosis of arrhythmogenic right ventricular cardiomyopathy/dysplasia: proposed modification of the Task Force Criteria. Eur Heart J 2010;31:806–14; with permission.

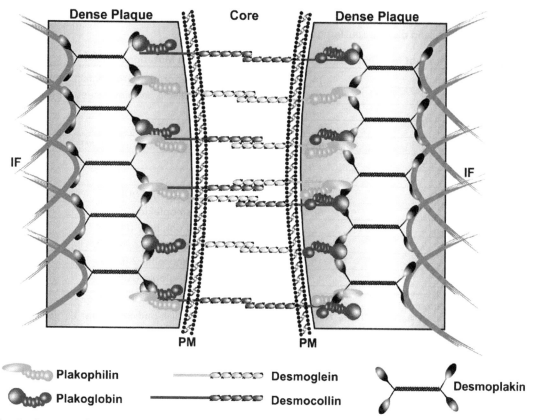

Fig. 2. The intracellular and intercellular components of the desmosomal plaque. Three separate families of proteins assemble to form desmosome: desmosomal cadherins (desmoglein and desmocollin), armadillo proteins (plakoglobin and plakophilin), and plakins (desmoplakin). The desmosomal cadherins present with extracellular domains that play a pivotal role in cell adhesion; whereas, the intracellular domain interacts with the armadillo proteins. Among the latter, plakophilin binds to the N-terminal domain of desmoplakin and the C-terminal of desmoplakin anchors desmin intermediate filaments. IF, intermediate filaments; PM, cytoplasmic membrane. (*Modified from* Basso C, Corrado D, Marcus FI, et al. Arrhythmogenic right ventricular cardiomyopathy. Lancet 2009;373:1289–30; with permission.)

myocytes at the intercalated discs, particularly under conditions of mechanical stress.[15] Subsequently, myocyte degeneration and death occur, and are followed by fibrofatty myocardial replacement. Rather than being a continuous process, ARVC progresses through bursts of myocardial damages (hot phases).[2,6,9] These findings are in keeping with the clinically silent course of the disease with sudden occurrence of life-threatening arrhythmias. Environmental factors, such as sport activity, may facilitate disease progression by worsening cell adhesion disruption.[2]

This pathogenic hypothesis is supported by studies using transgenic animal models. Heterozygous JUP-deficient mice showed RV dilation/dysfunction and ventricular arrhythmia.[36] In this study, endurance training accelerated the

development of RV dysfunction and arrhythmias. A transgenic mouse with cardiac-restricted over-expression of the C-terminal mutant (R2834H) DSP shows an increase myocardial apoptosis, fibrosis, and fatty replacement, as well as biventricular dilatation/dysfunction.[37] Garcia-Gras and colleagues[38] demonstrated that cardiac-specific loss of the DSP was sufficient to cause nuclear translocation of plakoglobin, increased expression of adipogenic and fibrogenic genes, and lead the development of an ARVC-like phenotype (myocardial fibrofatty replacement, cavity enlargement, and ventricular arrhythmia).

Further insights into the pathogenesis of ARVC were provided by the study of transgenic mice (Tg-NS) with cardiac overexpression of the DSG2 gene mutation.[39] Transgenic mice recapitulated the disease clinical features, including premature

Table 2
Chromosomal loci and disease-causing genes in ARVC

Designation (Pattern of Inheritance)	Chromosomal Locus	Gene Mutations
ARVD1 (AD)	14q23-q24	Transforming growth factor-β3 (TGFβ3)
ARVD2 (AD)	1q42-q43	Cardiac ryanodine receptor (RyR2)
ARVD3 (AD)	14q12-q22	?
ARVD4 (AD)	2q32.1-q32.3	?
ARVD5 (AD)	3p23	Transmembrane 43 (TMEM43)
ARVD6 (AD)	10p12-p14	?
ARVD7 (AD)	10q22	?
Naxos disease (AR)	17q21	Plakoglobin (JUP)
ARVD8 (AD)	6p24	Desmoplakin (DSP)
ARVD 9 (AD)	12p11	Plakophilin-2 (PKP2)
ARVD 10 (AD)	18q12.1	Desmoglein-2 (DSG2)
ARVD 11 (AD)	18q12.1	Desmocollin-2 (DSC2)
ARVD 12 (AD)	17q21	Plakoglobin (JUP)

Abbreviations: AD, autosomal dominant; AR, autosomal recessive.
Data from Corrado D, Basso C, Thiene G. Arrhythmogenic right ventricular cardiomyopathy: an update. Heart 2009;95:766–73.

sudden death, spontaneous ventricular arrhythmias, biventricular dilatation/dysplasia, and aneurysms. The study demonstrated for the first time that myocyte necrosis is the key initiator of myocardial injury, triggering progressive myocardial damage and atrophy with reactive myocarditis, followed by injury repair with fibrofatty tissue replacement.

Genetic Test for Diagnosis of ARVC

At present, a genetic confirmatory test for diagnosis of ARVC in sporadic cases is not routinely applicable in clinical practice. The clinical utility of molecular genetic study is limited to preclinical diagnosis of ARVC in the setting of a familial disease. Clinical manifestations of ARVC usually develop during adolescence and young adulthood, and are preceded by a long preclinical phase. Early ARVC diagnosis in family members with an affected proband offers the possibilities of focused management strategy consisting of lifestyle modifications (restriction from competitive sport), close clinical follow-up, and timely therapy (ie, AADs/ β-blockers, catheter ablation, and ICD) to prevent disease worsening and sudden death.[10,14]

Molecular Autopsy

Arrhythmic sudden death might occur in a preclinical stage of ARVC before diagnostic histopathologic features become evident at post mortem.

Therefore, diagnosis of the cause of death may depend on molecular genetic testing (molecular autopsy) with identification of a pathogenetic gene defect. The current role of molecular autopsy for ARVC in sudden cardiac death victims is limited, but would become crucial with better understanding of the molecular background of ARVC in the future.[40]

THERAPY
Risk Stratification

Mortality rate of patients with ARVC on medical therapy is estimated to be around 1% per year. Most of the deaths are related to arrhythmias, which can occur at any time during the disease course. The available data based on autopsy series or retrospective clinical studies suggest that young age, prior cardiac arrest, fast and poorly tolerated VT, syncope, severe RV dysfunction, LV involvement with heart failure and familial occurrence of juvenile sudden death are potential predictors of sudden death and worse outcome.[41]

Progressive ventricular dysfunction leading to heart failure and embolic stroke may cause death in a small proportion of patients.[6]

There are conflicting data on the prognostic values of electrophysiologic study (EPS) with programmed ventricular stimulation (PVS) in ARVC.[42–47] The largest study[43] reported that the incidence of appropriate ICD discharge did not differ in patients with and without inducible

VT/VF at PVS, regardless of indication for ICD implant. This finding is in agreement with the limitation of EPS for arrhythmic risk stratification of other nonischemic heart diseases, such as hypertrophic and dilated cardiomyopathy. In the study by Wichter and colleagues,[44] inducibility of VT or VF at preimplant EPS, in subjects with previous history of cardiac arrest or sustained VT, demonstrated a trend toward statistical significance for subsequent appropriate device interventions. Roguin and colleagues[42] reported that VT induction was the most significant independent predictor of appropriate ICD firing in their cohort of subjects with ARVC.

Further studies on a larger subject population over a longer follow-up are needed to conclusively determine the value of PVS for risk stratification of patients with ARVC patients.

Drug Therapy

AAD therapy is the first-line treatment for patients with ARVC with well-tolerated and nonlife-threatening ventricular arrhythmias. Sotalol has been frequently used for prevention of ventricular arrhythmia or the reduction of ICD intervention.[48,49] Amiodarone alone or in combination with β-blocker has been reported as an alternative approach, although potentially dangerous cardiac and noncardiac side effects should be taken into account.

The largest European experience with acute and long-term efficacy of AAD therapy was published in 1992[48] and updated in 2005.[49] The efficacy of AAD was determined by PVS for inducible VT and by exercise test/24-hour Holter monitoring for noninducible VT. Sotalol was the most effective drug with an overall success rate of 68%.

On the contrary, a North American study showed that sotalol did not result in a significantly longer ICD-shock free survival in subjects with ARVC.[50] Instead, amiodarone guaranteed greater success rate for prevention of ventricular arrhythmias. Of note, unlike the previous reports,[51,52] this study did not show a protective effect of β-blocker.

The current evidence suggests that asymptomatic individuals should be included in a follow-up program with noninvasive evaluation on a regular basis for early identification of warning symptoms and demonstration of disease progression or ventricular arrhythmias.

Whether prophylactic use of β-blocker, AADs, and angiotensin-converting enzyme (ACE) inhibitors/angiotensin receptor blocker may reduce arrhythmic complications and disease progression in asymptomatic patients or gene carriers remains to be proven.[42,45,50]

In patients with RV or biventricular heart failure, treatment consists of diuretics, ACE inhibitors/angiotensin receptor blocker and digitalis, as well as anticoagulants.

Catheter Ablation

The main mechanism of VT in ARVC is scar-related reentry. The arrhythmogenic substrate consists of myocardial atrophy with fibrofatty replacement. Three-dimensional (3D) electroanatomical mapping by CARTO system (CARTO, BiosenseWebster, Diamond Bar, CA, USA) offers the possibility to delineate electroanatomical scar, which corresponds to areas of low amplitude and fractionated intracardiac electrograms. Three-dimensional mapping tools are used to perform substrate-based ablations for VT, which is hemodynamically not tolerated or not inducible.[53–58]

Once the reentry circuit is demonstrated using activation or substrate mapping, its interruption across the critical isthmus is achieved by a linear ablation lesion connecting or encircling electrical scar areas. Deeper and transmural lesion may be obtained by using irrigation catheters with improvement of the ablation success rates.[54,56,59]

Several studies investigated acute- and long-term efficacy of catheter ablation of VT in ARVC (**Table 3**).

Marchlinski and colleagues[54] reported the acute and long-term success rates of substrate-guided VT ablation. Complete acute success (no inducible VT) was achieved in 14 of 19 subjects (74%) and partial success in the remaining 5 subjects. During a 27-month follow-up, 17 of 19 subjects (84%) were free from VT recurrence. Of note, more than one procedure was required in 13 of 19 subjects (68%). The efficacies of catheter ablation guided by CARTO system was confirmed by subsequent studies.[53,55–57] Yao and colleagues[58] also obtained good acute (75%) and long-term success rate (81% at 29 months of follow-up) using EnSite system (EnSite, St Jude Medical Inc, St Paul, MN, USA), which is another 3-D mapping tool.

Nogami and colleagues[60] reported a substrate-based approach of catheter ablation guided by an isolated delayed component, which was defined as a ventricular electrogram after the QRS separated by greater than or equal to 40 milliseconds or a low amplitude signal of less than 0.1 mV. They concluded that changes of isolated delayed components at the ablation target site induced by radiofrequency current, reflected modifications of the arrhythmogenic substrate, was associated with a favorable long-term outcome.

Unsatisfactory long-term results have been reported by the other studies. Dalal and colleagues[61]

Table 3
Results of VT catheter ablation in ARVC

Study, Year	Ref	Subjects (n)	Complete Success % (Partial)	Mapping	Irrigation Catheter	Suspected Epicardial VT	Complications	ICD (%)	F/U (months)	VT Rec (%)	F/U Death
Garcia et al, 2009[a]	62	13	85 (92)	CARTO	yes	[a]	0	92	18	23	1 HT
Nogami et al, 2008	60	18	45 (67)	CARTO[b]	no	2/18	0	33	61	33	2 HF, 1NC
Dalal et al, 2007	61	24	46 (77)	CARTO[b]	no	NA	1 death	79	32	83	2 HT
Yao et al, 2007	58	32	75	NCM	yes	NA	0	6	29	19	0
Satomi st al, 2006	57	17	88	CARTO	no	4/13	0	12	26	24	0
Verma et al, 2005	56	22	82 (95)	CARTO	yes	NA	1 tamponade	100	37	36	0
Miljoen et al, 2005	55	11	73	CARTO	no	4/12	0	64	20	45	1NC
Marchlinski et al, 2004	54	19	74 (100)	CARTO	yes	NA	0	74	27	11	0
O'Donnell et al, 2003	59	17	48 (70)	no	yes	NA	NA	47	58	47	0
Reithmann et al, 2003	53	5	40 (80)	CARTO	no	4/5	0	80	7	20	0

Abbreviations: F/U, follow-up; HF, heart failure; HT, heart transplant; NA, not available; NC, noncardiac death; NCM, noncontact mapping; Rec, recurrence; Ref, reference number.
[a] Epicardial mapping was done in all subjects.
[b] CARTO system was rarely used.

showed that 85% of ablation procedures were followed by VT relapses. Verma and colleagues[56] reported a recurrence rate of 47% during 3 years and Nogami and colleagues[60] of 49% during 5 years of follow-up.

This high incidence of VT relapses has been ascribed to the progressive nature of the disease, which creates new arrhythmogenic substrates over time. Moreover, the possible epicardial location of arrhythmogenic substrate may partially, explain the failure of traditional endocardial mapping/catheter ablation. The possible epicardial location of the reentry circuit reflects the propensity of the wave front lesion to progress from the epicardium to the endocardium.[2] Recently, the feasibility of epicardial catheter ablation has been reported.[62] Thirteen subjects with ARVC underwent epicardial mapping and VT ablation after previously failed endocardial procedures. The extent of the low voltage areas (electroanatomical scar) was larger on the epicardial site of the RV wall than on the endocardium. Complete success was achieved in 11 of 13 subjects (85%) and partial success in 12 of 13 subjects (92%). During 18 months of follow-up, 10 of 13 subjects (77%) were free of VT.

Because of the high rate of late VT recurrence and the periprocedural risk of complications (also potentially life threatening),[56,61] catheter ablation of VT in patients with ARVC should be considered as a palliative therapy approach and reserved for patients with drug refractory incessant VT or frequent VT recurrences requiring ICD intervention.

Implantable Cardioverter Defibrillator

Data from observational studies on a large population of patients with ARVC have established the efficacy and safety of ICD therapy. Five major studies[42–47] on ICD therapy are summarized in **Table 4**.

Corrado and colleagues[43] published the largest multicenter experience of ICD therapy (132 subjects with ARVC). Approximately 50% of the 132 study subjects had at least 1 appropriate ICD intervention during a mean 3.3 years of follow-up, despite AADs therapy. Furthermore, 24% of the total subject population experienced greater than or equal to 1 episode of VF or ventricular flutter, documented by the stored intracardiac ECG, that in all likelihood would have been fatal in the absence of device therapy (**Fig. 3**). Analysis of risk factors showed that younger age, history of cardiac arrest or hemodynamically unstable VT, and LV involvement were independent clinical variables associated with the occurrence of such life-threatening arrhythmias. On the contrary, therapy

with ICD did not improve survival in the subgroup of subjects presenting with hemodynamically stable monomorphic VT.

Wichter and colleagues[44] reported a single-center experience of ICD therapy in 60 subjects with ARVC during follow-up of 80±43 months. The majority of subjects received an ICD for secondary prevention (93%). The study confirmed the life-saving role of ICD therapy in high-risk subgroups of patients with ARVC. However, 37 of 60 subjects (62%) had a total of 53 adverse events. In other studies, the rate of ICD-related complications was reported to range from 10% to 62%.[42–47]

Inappropriate ICD intervention is also a serious problem and occurs in 10% to 25% of patients with ARVC with ICD caused by sinus tachycardia, atrial tachyarrhythmia, oversensing, or lead failure.[42–47] Careful attention should be paid to reduce the incidence of inappropriate ICD discharge by appropriate ICD programming or administration of β-blocker.

Current Indications for ICD Implantation

Patients with prior cardiac arrest and those with hemodynamically unstable VT carry the highest risk of sudden death and benefit of ICD implantation (secondary prevention). In this high-risk group of patients, the rate of appropriate ICD intervention against life-threatening ventricular arrhythmias (that in all likelihood would have been fatal in the absence of shock therapy) is approximately 8% to 10% per year and the estimated mortality reduction at 36 months of follow-up ranges from 24% to 35%.[43–46] On the contrary, ICD implantation for primary prevention is unjustified in the general ARVC population. As indicated by a recent multicenter study[47] on prophylactic device implantation in subjects with ARVC with no sustained VT or VF, asymptomatic probands and relatives may not benefit from ICD therapy, regardless of family history of sudden death or inducibility at PVS. This patient cohort carries a low arrhythmic risk over a long-term follow-up (ICD intervention rate <1 per year), in addition to a significant rate of device-related complications and inappropriate discharges.[42–47] Patients with hemodynamically tolerated sustained VT or nonsustained on Holter or exercise testing have an intermediate arrhythmic risk (ICD intervention rate approximately 1%–2% per year). In this patient subgroup, the decision regarding ICD therapy needs to be individualized; AADs therapy (including β-blockers) or catheter ablation seem to be reasonable first-line therapies. Whether, in the absence of syncope or significant ventricular arrhythmias, severe dilatation or

Table 4
ICD therapy in subjects with ARVC

Study	Ref	Year	Subjects	Primary (%)	F/U (Months)	Appropriate ICD Therapy (%)	Inappropriate ICD Therapy (%)	Life Saving (%)	Mortality (%)	Transplant (n)	Complication (%)
Corrado et al	[43]	2003	132	22	39 ± 25	48	16	24	3	1	14
Wichter et al	[44]	2004	60	7	80 ± 43	68	23	40	13	2	62
Rougin et al	[42]	2004	42	40	42 ± 26	78	25	NA	2	1	14
Hdgkinson et al	[45]	2005	48	73	31	70	10	30	0	3	6
Piccini et al	[46]	2005	67[a]	42	48 ± 32	66	24	21	4	2	14
Corrado et al	[47]	2010	106	100	58 ± 35	24	19	16	0	0	17

Abbreviations: F/U, follow-up; NA, not available; Ref, reference number.
[a] This study included 55 definite and 12 probable subjects with ARVC and 38 subjects were also included in prior study.[42]

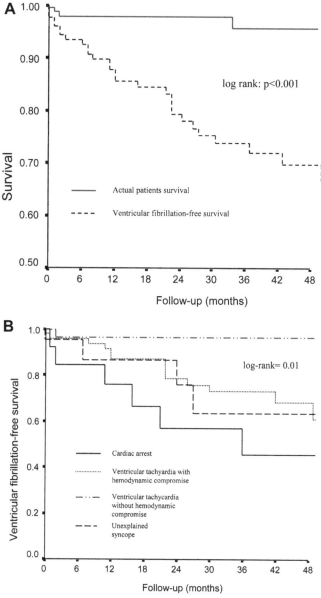

Fig. 3. (*A*) Kaplan-Meier analysis of actual subject survival (*upper line*) compared with survival free of ventricular fibrillation (*lower line*) that in all likelihood would have been fatal in the absence of an implantable cardioverter-defibrillator. The divergence between the lines reflects the estimated mortality reduction by ICD therapy of 24% at 3 years of follow-up. (*B*) Kaplan-Meier curves of freedom from ICD interventions on VF for different subject subgroups stratified for clinical presentation. Subjects who received an ICD because of sustained VT without hemodynamic compromise had a significantly lower incidence of VF during follow-up. (*Modified from* Corrado D, Leoni L, Link MS, et al. Implantable cardioverter-defibrillator therapy for prevention of sudden death in patients with arrhythmogenic right ventricular cardiomyopathy/dysplasia. Circulation 2003;108:3084–91; with permission.)

dysfunction of RV, LV, or both, as well as early onset of structurally severe disease (aged <35 years) require prophylactic ICD remain to be determined.

SUMMARY

In the future, clinical studies on larger cohorts for patients who have ARVC with longer follow-up will provide further data on genetic background, accuracy of diagnostic criteria, stratification of arrhythmic risk, and efficacy of therapeutic interventions.

ACKNOWLEDGMENTS

This work was supported by the Ministry of Health, Rome; Fondazione Cariparo, Padova and Rovigo; and Registry of Cardio-Cerebro-Vascular Pathology, Veneto Region, Venice, Italy.

REFERENCES

1. Thiene G, Nava A, Corrado D, et al. Right ventricular cardiomyopathy and sudden death in young people. N Engl J Med 1988;318:129–33.
2. Basso C, Corrado D, Marcus FI, et al. Arrhythmogenic right ventricular cardiomyopathy. Lancet 2009;373:1289–300.
3. Basso C, Thiene G, Corrado D, et al. Arrhythmogenic right ventricular cardiomyopathy. dysplasia, dystrophy, or myocarditis? Circulation 1996;94:983–91.
4. Corrado D, Basso C, Thiene G, et al. Spectrum of clinicopathologic manifestations of arrhythmogenic right ventricular cardiomyopathy/dysplasia: a multicenter study. J Am Coll Cardiol 1997;30:1512–20.
5. Corrado D, Basso C, Thiene G. Arrhythmogenic right ventricular cardiomyopathy: diagnosis, prognosis, and treatment. Heart 2000;83:588–95.
6. Corrado D, Basso C, Thiene G. Arrhythmogenic right ventricular cardiomyopathy: an update. Heart 2009;95:766–73.
7. Corrado D, Basso C, Schiavon M, et al. Screening for hypertrophic cardiomyopathy in young athletes. N Engl J Med 1998;339:364–9.
8. Corrado D, Basso C, Pavei A, et al. Trends in sudden cardiovascular death in young competitive athletes after implementation of a preparticipation screening program. JAMA 2006;296:1593–601.
9. Sen-Chowdhry S, Syrris P, McKenna WJ. Genetics of right ventricular cardiomyopathy. J Cardiovasc Electrophysiol 2005;16:927–35.
10. Corrado D, Thiene G. Arrhythmogenic right ventricular cardiomyopathy/dysplasia: clinical impact of molecular genetic studies. Circulation 2006;113:1634–7.
11. Sen-Chowdhry S, Syrris P, McKenna WJ. Role of genetic analysis in the management of patients with arrhythmogenic right ventricular dysplasia/cardiomyopathy. J Am Coll Cardiol 2007;50:1813–21.
12. McKenna WJ, Thiene G, Nava A, et al. Diagnosis of arrhythmogenic right ventricular dysplasia/cardiomyopathy. Task force of the working group myocardial and pericardial disease of the european society of cardiology and of the scientific council on cardiomyopathies of the international society and federation of cardiology. Br Heart J 1994;71:215–8.
13. Marcus FI, McKenna WJ, Sherrill D, et al. Diagnosis of arrhythmogenic right ventricular cardiomyopathy/dysplasia: proposed modification of the task force criteria. Eur Heart J 2010;31:806–14.
14. Nava A, Bauce B, Basso C, et al. Clinical profile and long-term follow-up of 37 families with arrhythmogenic right ventricular cardiomyopathy. J Am Coll Cardiol 2000;36:2226–33.
15. McKoy G, Protonotarios N, Crosby A, et al. Identification of a deletion in plakoglobin in arrhythmogenic right ventricular cardiomyopathy with palmoplantar keratoderma and woolly hair (Naxos disease). Lancet 2000;355:2119–24.
16. Norgett EE, Hatsell SJ, Carvajal-Huerta L, et al. Recessive mutation in desmoplakin disrupts desmoplakin-intermediate filament interactions and causes dilated cardiomyopathy, woolly hair and keratoderma. Hum Mol Genet 2000;9:2761–6.
17. Nava A, Canciani B, Buja G, et al. Electrovectorcardiographic study of negative T waves on precordial leads in arrhythmogenic right ventricular dysplasia: relationship with right ventricular volumes. J Electrocardiol 1988;21:239–45.
18. Nasir K, Bomma C, Tandri H, et al. Electrocardiographic features of arrhythmogenic right ventricular dysplasia/cardiomyopathy according to disease severity: a need to broaden diagnostic criteria. Circulation 2004;110:1527–34.
19. Cox MG, Nelen MR, Wilde AA, et al. Activation delay and VT parameters in arrhythmogenic right ventricular dysplasia/cardiomyopathy: toward improvement of diagnostic ECG criteria. J Cardiovasc Electrophysiol 2008;19:775–81.
20. Nava A, Folino AF, Bauce B, et al. Signal-averaged electrocardiogram in patients with arrhythmogenic right ventricular cardiomyopathy and ventricular arrhythmias. Eur Heart J 2000;21:58–65.
21. Turrini P, Corrado D, Basso C, et al. Dispersion of ventricular depolarization-repolarization: a noninvasive marker for risk stratification in arrhythmogenic right ventricular cardiomyopathy. Circulation 2001;103:3075–80.
22. Marcus FI, Fontaine GH, Guiraudon G, et al. Right ventricular dysplasia: a report of 24 adult cases. Circulation 1982;65:384–98.
23. Nava A, Thiene G, Canciani B, et al. Familial occurrence of right ventricular dysplasia: a study involving nine families. J Am Coll Cardiol 1988;12:1222–8.
24. Rampazzo A, Nava A, Danieli GA, et al. The gene for arrhythmogenic right ventricular cardiomyopathy maps to chromosome 14q23–q24. Hum Mol Genet 1994;3:959–62.

25. Gerull B, Heuser A, Wichter T, et al. Mutations in the desmosomal protein plakophilin-2 are common in arrhythmogenic right ventricular cardiomyopathy. Nat Genet 2004;36:1162–4.

26. Dalal D, Molin LH, Piccini J, et al. Clinical features of arrhythmogenic right ventricular dysplasia/cardiomyopathy associated with mutations in plakophilin-2. Circulation 2006;113:1641–9.

27. van Tintelen JP, Entius MM, Bhuiyan ZA, et al. Plakophilin-2 mutations are the major determinant of familial arrhythmogenic right ventricular dysplasia/cardiomyopathy. Circulation 2006;113:1650–8.

28. Pilichou K, Nava A, Basso C, et al. Mutations in desmoglein-2 gene are associated with arrhythmogenic right ventricular cardiomyopathy. Circulation 2006;113:1171–9.

29. Awad MM, Dalal D, Cho E, et al. DSG2 mutations contribute to arrhythmogenic right ventricular dysplasia/cardiomyopathy. Am J Hum Genet 2006; 79:136–42.

30. Syrris P, Ward D, Evans A, et al. Arrhythmogenic right ventricular dysplasia/cardiomyopathy associated with mutations in the desmosomal gene desmocollin-2. Am J Hum Genet 2006;79:978–84.

31. Heuser A, Plovie ER, Ellinor PT, et al. Mutant desmocollin-2 causes arrhythmogenic right ventricular cardiomyopathy. Am J Hum Genet 2006;79: 1081–8.

32. Awad MM, Calkins H, Judge DP. Mechanisms of disease: molecular genetics of arrhythmogenic right ventricular dysplasia/cardiomyopathy. Nat Clin Pract Cardiovasc Med 2008;5:258–67.

33. Tiso N, Stephan DA, Nava A, et al. Identification of mutations in the cardiac ryanodine receptor gene in families affected with arrhythmogenic right ventricular cardiomyopathy type 2 (ARVD2). Hum Mol Genet 2001;10:189–94.

34. Beffagna G, Occhi G, Nava A, et al. Regulatory mutations in transforming growth factor-beta3 gene cause arrhythmogenic right ventricular cardiomyopathy type 1. Cardiovasc Res 2005;65:366–73.

35. Merner ND, Hodgkinson KA, Haywood AF, et al. Arrhythmogenic right ventricular cardiomyopathy type 5 is a fully penetrant, lethal arrhythmic disorder caused by a missense mutation in the TMEM43 gene. Am J Hum Genet 2008;82:809–21.

36. Kirchhof P, Fabritz L, Zwiener M, et al. Age- and training-dependent development of arrhythmogenic right ventricular cardiomyopathy in heterozygous plakoglobin-deficient mice. Circulation 2006;114: 1799–806.

37. Yang Z, Bowles NE, Scherer SE, et al. Desmosomal dysfunction due to mutations in desmoplakin causes arrhythmogenic right ventricular dysplasia/cardiomyopathy. Circ Res 2006;99:646–55.

38. Garcia-Gras E, Lombardi R, Giocondo MJ, et al. Suppression of canonical Wnt/beta-catenin signaling by nuclear plakoglobin recapitulates phenotype of arrhythmogenic right ventricular cardiomyopathy. J Clin Invest 2006;116:2012–21.

39. Pilichou K, Remme CA, Basso C, et al. Myocyte necrosis underlies progressive myocardial dystrophy in mouse dsg2-related arrhythmogenic right ventricular cardiomyopathy. J Exp Med 2009; 206:1787–802.

40. Basso C, Carturan E, Pilichou K, et al. Sudden cardiac death with normal heart molecular autopsy. Cardiovasc Pathol 2010. [Epub ahead of print].

41. Buja G, Estes NA 3rd, Wichter T, et al. Arrhythmogenic right ventricular cardiomyopathy/dysplasia: risk stratification and therapy. Prog Cardiovasc Dis 2008;50:282–93.

42. Roguin A, Bomma CS, Nasir K, et al. Implantable cardioverter-defibrillators in patients with arrhythmogenic right ventricular dysplasia/cardiomyopathy. J Am Coll Cardiol 2004;43:1843–52.

43. Corrado D, Leoni L, Link MS, et al. Implantable cardioverter-defibrillator therapy for prevention of sudden death in patients with arrhythmogenic right ventricular cardiomyopathy/dysplasia. Circulation 2003;108:3084–91.

44. Wichter T, Paul M, Wollmann C, et al. Implantable cardioverter/defibrillator therapy in arrhythmogenic right ventricular cardiomyopathy: single-center experience of long-term follow-up and complications in 60 patients. Circulation 2004;109:1503–8.

45. Hodgkinson KA, Parfrey PS, Bassett AS, et al. The impact of implantable cardioverter-defibrillator therapy on survival in autosomal-dominant arrhythmogenic right ventricular cardiomyopathy (ARVD5). J Am Coll Cardiol 2005;45:400–8.

46. Piccini JP, Dalal D, Roguin A, et al. Predictors of appropriate implantable defibrillator therapies in patients with arrhythmogenic right ventricular dysplasia. Heart Rhythm 2005;2:1188–94.

47. Corrado D, Calkins H, Link MS, et al. Prophylactic implantable defibrillator in patients with arrhythmogenic right ventricular cardiomyopathy/dysplasia and no prior ventricular fibrillation or sustained ventricular tachycardia. Circulation 2010;122: 1144–52.

48. Wichter T, Borggrefe M, Haverkamp W, et al. Efficacy of antiarrhythmic drugs in patients with arrhythmogenic right ventricular disease. Results in patients with inducible and noninducible ventricular tachycardia. Circulation 1992;86:29–37.

49. Wichter T, Paul TM, Eckardt L, et al. Arrhythmogenic right ventricular cardiomyopathy. Antiarrhythmic drugs, catheter ablation, or ICD? Herz 2005;30:91–101.

50. Marcus GM, Glidden DV, Polonsky B, et al. Efficacy of antiarrhythmic drugs in arrhythmogenic right ventricular cardiomyopathy: a report from the North American ARVC Registry. J Am Coll Cardiol 2009; 54:609–15.

51. Calkins H. Arrhythmogenic right-ventricular dysplasia/cardiomyopathy. Curr Opin Cardiol 2006;21:55–63.

52. Sen-Chowdhry S, Lowe MD, Sporton SC, et al. Arrhythmogenic right ventricular cardiomyopathy: clinical presentation, diagnosis, and management. Am J Med 2004;117:685–95.

53. Reithmann C, Hahnefeld A, Remp T, et al. Electroanatomic mapping of endocardial right ventricular activation as a guide for catheter ablation in patients with arrhythmogenic right ventricular dysplasia. Pacing Clin Electrophysiol 2003;26:1308–16.

54. Marchlinski FE, Zado E, Dixit S, et al. Electroanatomic substrate and outcome of catheter ablative therapy for ventricular tachycardia in setting of right ventricular cardiomyopathy. Circulation 2004;110: 2293–8.

55. Miljoen H, State S, de Chillou C, et al. Electroanatomic mapping characteristics of ventricular tachycardia in patients with arrhythmogenic right ventricular cardiomyopathy/dysplasia. Europace 2005;7:516–24.

56. Verma A, Kilicaslan F, Schweikert RA, et al. Short- and long-term success of substrate-based mapping and ablation of ventricular tachycardia in arrhythmogenic right ventricular dysplasia. Circulation 2005;111:3209–16.

57. Satomi K, Kurita T, Suyama K, et al. Catheter ablation of stable and unstable ventricular tachycardias in patients with arrhythmogenic right ventricular dysplasia. J Cardiovasc Electrophysiol 2006;17: 469–76.

58. Yao Y, Zhang S, He DS, et al. Radiofrequency ablation of the ventricular tachycardia with arrhythmogenic right ventricular cardiomyopathy using non-contact mapping. Pacing Clin Electrophysiol 2007;30: 526–33.

59. O'Donnell D, Cox D, Bourke J, et al. Clinical and electrophysiological differences between patients with arrhythmogenic right ventricular dysplasia and right ventricular outflow tract tachycardia. Eur Heart J 2003;24:801–10.

60. Nogami A, Sugiyasu A, Tada H, et al. Changes in the isolated delayed component as an endpoint of catheter ablation in arrhythmogenic right ventricular cardiomyopathy: predictor for long-term success. J Cardiovasc Electrophysiol 2008;19:681–8.

61. Dalal D, Jain R, Tandri H, et al. Long-term efficacy of catheter ablation of ventricular tachycardia in patients with arrhythmogenic right ventricular dysplasia/cardiomyopathy. J Am Coll Cardiol 2007; 50:432–40.

62. Garcia FC, Bazan V, Zado ES, et al. Epicardial substrate and outcome with epicardial ablation of ventricular tachycardia in arrhythmogenic right ventricular cardiomyopathy/dysplasia. Circulation 2009;120:366–75.

Hypertrophic Cardiomyopathy

Christopher Critoph, BM, Perry Elliott, MBBS, MD*

KEYWORDS

- Hypertrophic cardiomyopathy • Sudden death
- Sarcomere proteins • Heart failure • Stroke • Arrhythmia

Cardiomyopathies are myocardial disorders in which the heart is structurally and functionally abnormal, in the absence of coronary artery disease, valvular heart disease, hypertension, or congenital heart disease sufficient to cause the observed myocardial abnormality.[1] Cardiomyopathies are classified into 4 main subtypes, based on ventricular morphology and physiology; hypertrophic cardiomyopathy (HCM) is defined as left ventricular (LV) hypertrophy in the absence of abnormal loading conditions sufficient to explain the degree of hypertrophy.[1]

HCM is the commonest inherited cardiac disease, with a population prevalence of approximately 1 in 500.[2] In most adolescents and adults, HCM is inherited as an autosomal dominant trait caused by mutations in cardiac sarcomere protein genes.[3–5] A smaller number are caused by syndromic disorders such as Noonan and LEOPARD (lentigines, electrocardiograph [ECG] abnormalities, ocular hypertelorism, pulmonary stenosis, abnormalities of the genitalia, retardation of growth, and deafness), or inherited metabolic diseases such as glycogen and lysosomal storage disorders (**Table 1**).

In some series, HCM is the most common cause of sudden death in young people,[6,7] but most patients are asymptomatic and therefore often remain undiagnosed. Long-term, many patients develop progressive symptoms caused by gradual deterioration in LV function. This so-called end stage is characterized by severe impairment of contractile performance and is associated with a poor prognosis.[8] Diastolic function is impaired in most patients and may in some individuals so dominate the clinical picture that it resembles restrictive cardiomyopathy.[9]

GENETICS

In 50% to 60% of individuals, HCM is inherited as an autosomal dominant trait caused by mutations in genes that encode proteins of the cardiac sarcomere; the commonest are β-myosin heavy chain, cardiac troponin T, cardiac troponin I, α-tropomyosin, cardiac myosin binding protein C, the essential and regulatory myosin light chains, and cardiac actin. Other genes, such as those encoding α-myosin, titin, and proteins of the Z-disc, account for less than 1% of cases.[10]

Given the extent of genetic heterogeneity and the variable effect of different mutations on the structure and function of individual peptides, HCM is characterized by marked heterogeneity in disease severity and outcomes. For example, most disease-causing mutations in β-myosin heavy chain gene are found in 1 of 4 locations: the actin binding site, the nucleotide binding pocket, a region adjacent to the binding site for 2 reactive thiols in the hinge region, and the α-helix close to the essential light chain interaction site. Thus, depending on the position of the mutation, changes would be predicted in ATPase activity, actin-myosin interaction, and protein conformation during contraction. However, the clinical manifestations of identical mutations are highly variable, even within the same family, indicating that other genetic and possibly environmental factors influence disease expression. Evidence from murine models suggests that genetic background can modify the

The authors have nothing to disclose.
The Heart Hospital, 16–18 Westmoreland Street, London, W1G 8PH, UK
* Corresponding author.
E-mail address: perry.elliott@ucl.ac.uk

Table 1
Classification and causes of HCM

Familial	Nonfamilial
Familial, unknown gene	Obesity
Sarcomeric protein disease	Infants of diabetic mothers
β-Myosin heavy chain	Athletic training
Cardiac myosin binding protein C	Amyloid (AL/prealbumin)
Cardiac troponin I	
Troponin T	
α-Tropomyosin	
Essential myosin light chain	
Regulatory myosin light chain	
Cardiac actin	
α-Myosin heavy chain	
Titin	
Troponin C	
Muscle LIM protein	
Glycogen storage disease	
(eg, GSD II [Pompe disease]; GSD III [Forbes disease], AMP kinase [WPW, HCM, conduction disease])	
Danon disease	
Lysosomal storage diseases	
(eg, Anderson-Fabry disease, Hurler syndrome)	
Disorders of fatty acid metabolism	
Carnitine deficiency	
Phosphorylase B kinase deficiency	
Mitochondrial cytopathies	
(eg, MELAS, MERRF, LHON)	
Syndromic HCM	
• Noonan syndrome	
• LEOPARD syndrome	
• Friedreich ataxia	
• Beckwith-Wiedermann syndrome	
• Swyer syndrome (pure gonadal dysgenesis)	
• Costello syndrome	
Other:	
• Phospholamban promoter	
• Familial amyloid	

Abbreviations: GSD, glycogen storage disease; LEOPARD, lentigines, electrocardiograph abnormalities, ocular hypertelorism, pulmonary stenosis, abnormalities of the genitalia, retardation of growth, and deafness; LHON, Leber hereditary optic neuropathy; MELAS, mitochondrial encephalopathy, lactic acidosis, and strokelike episodes; MERRF, myoclonic epilepsy with ragged red fibers; WPW, Wolff-Parkinson-White syndrome.

Data from Elliott P, Andersson B, Arbustini E, et al. Classification of the cardiomyopathies: a position statement from the European Society of Cardiology working group on myocardial and pericardial diseases. Eur Heart J 2008;29:273.

hypertrophic phenotype. Some studies have suggested that common genetic polymorphisms in genes important in the renin-angiotensin-aldosterone system, the androgen receptor, estrogen receptor 1 and 2 (ESR1/2), aromatase (CYP19A1) and endothelin-2 (*EDN2*) might exert minor effects on the clinical phenotype.[11–13]

Several malformation syndromes, most of which present in childhood, are associated with HCM. Noonan syndrome is characterized by short stature, dysmorphic facies, skeletal malformations, and a webbed neck.[14,15] Cardiac involvement, in the form of pulmonary valve stenosis and HCM, is present in up to 90% of patients.[16] Noonan syndrome can present with congestive cardiac failure in infancy and is frequently associated with biventricular hypertrophy and bilateral ventricular outflow tract obstruction.[16] Noonan syndrome is inherited as a genetically heterogeneous autosomal dominant trait with variable penetrance and expression. Most mutations affect genes important in the RAS-ERK pathway, specifically PTPN11,[17] SOS1,[18,19] and KRAS.[20–22] To date, at least 39 different mutations have been identified, accounting for approximately 50% of cases of Noonan syndrome.[14] Most patients with LEOPARD syndrome, which shares many phenotypic features with Noonan syndrome, have mutations in the PTPN11 gene.[23]

Many inherited inborn errors of metabolism are associated with LV hypertrophy. In adults, the most important is Anderson-Fabry disease, an X-linked dominant lysosomal storage disorder caused by mutations in the α-galactosidase A gene that causes progressive accumulation of glycosphingolipid in the skin, nervous system, kidneys, and heart.[24] Cardiac manifestations include progressive LV hypertrophy, valve disease, conduction abnormalities, and supraventricular and ventricular arrhythmias. Treatment with recombinant α-galactosidase A improves renal, neurologic, and cardiac manifestations.

Danon disease is an X-linked lysosomal storage disorder caused by mutations in the gene encoding the lysosome-associated membrane protein-2 (LAMP-2).[25] It is characterized by cardiomyopathy, skeletal myopathy, developmental delay, and intracytoplasmic accumulation of autophagic material and glycogen within vacuoles in cardiac and skeletal myocytes.[26] Men present in childhood and adolescence, whereas women develop hypertrophic and dilated cardiomyopathy during adulthood.[27] The prognosis is generally poor, with most patients dying from cardiac failure and, less commonly, sudden cardiac death. Other features of Danon disease include Wolff-Parkinson-White syndrome, increased serum creatine kinase and retinitis pigmentosa.

Pompe disease (glycogen storage disease type IIa) is an autosomal recessive disorder caused by a deficiency in the enzyme acid maltase.[28] Infantile, juvenile and adult variants are recognized, but only the infantile and childhood forms are characterized by myocardial glycogen deposition, massive cardiac hypertrophy and heart failure. Without treatment, the infantile form is usually fatal before 2 years of age because of cardiorespiratory failure. The ECG typically shows broad high-voltage QRS complexes and ventricular preexcitation.[29]

Mutations in the gene encoding the γ2 subunit of the adenosine monophosphate-activated protein kinase (PRKAG2)[30] are responsible for a syndrome of HCM, conduction system disease and Wolff-Parkinson-White syndrome. Histologically, there is accumulation of glycogen within cardiac myocytes and conduction tissue and excess mitochondria and ragged red fibers in skeletal muscle.[31] Patients develop progressive conduction disease, and LV hypertrophy and atrial arrhythmias are common.

Primary respiratory chain diseases caused by sporadic or inherited mutations in nuclear or mitochondrial DNA are rare causes of cardiomyopathy. Clinically, respiratory chain diseases vary in age at onset, symptoms, and the range and severity of organ involvement. In children, cardiac involvement (usually HCM) is present in up to 40% of mitochondrial encephalomyopathies.[32] Rapid progression to heart failure and sudden arrhythmic death is common in childhood presentations.[32,33]

Friedreich's ataxia is an autosomal recessive condition caused by mutations in the frataxin gene.[34] Cardiac involvement is common, and is usually characterized by concentric LV hypertrophy without LV outflow tract obstruction (LVOTO).[35] Progression to LV dilatation and heart failure is described,[36] but prognosis is usually determined by the neuromuscular disease.

PATHOLOGY

The macroscopic and histologic phenotype varies with the underlying genetic cause. The most common appearance is asymmetric septal hypertrophy, but any pattern of LV hypertrophy can be seen. Microscopically, HCM is characterized by a triad of myocyte hypertrophy, myocyte disarray (architectural disorganization of the myocardium, with adjacent myocytes aligned obliquely or perpendicular to one another), and interstitial fibrosis.[37,38] Small intramural coronary arteries are often dysplastic and narrowed because of wall thickening by smooth muscle cell hyperplasia.[39]

CLINICAL FEATURES OF HCM
Symptoms

Most patients with HCM complain of no symptoms. Some experience chest pain, breathlessness, fatigue, and palpitations, often with marked day-to-day variation. Syncope is also common and can be caused by many mechanisms including LVOTO, hypotension secondary to abnormal vascular responses, and arrhythmias.[40,41] Changes in LV loading conditions during exercise, heavy meals, and dehydration often precipitate symptoms.

Physical Examination

The cardiovascular examination in most patients is normal. In some, the jugular venous pulsation may have a prominent a wave, caused by reduced right ventricular compliance. The LV impulse is typically sustained, or double, reflecting an atrial impulse followed by LV contraction. LVOTO causes a rapid upstroke and downstroke to the arterial pulse, occasionally followed by a palpable reflected wave, resulting in a bisferiens pulse. On auscultation, LVOTO causes a harsh ejection systolic murmur at the left sternal edge, which increases in intensity during strain phase of the Valsalva or when standing from the squatting position. Most patients with LVOTO also have mitral regurgitation (caused by abnormal coaptation of the mitral valve leaflets during systole). This regurgitation causes a pansystolic, high-frequency murmur at the apex, radiating to the axilla. A third or fourth heart sound is common.

DIAGNOSTIC TESTS
Electrocardiography

The resting 12-lead ECG is abnormal in 95% of patients with HCM. The commonest abnormalities are ventricular hypertrophy, repolarization abnormalities, pathologic Q waves, and left atrial enlargement. Giant negative T waves in the mid-precordial leads are characteristic of apical HCM.[42] A short PR interval without ventricular pre-excitation is common.[43] Atrioventricular conduction delay (including first-degree block) is rare except in particular subtypes of HCM (eg, PRKAG2 mutations and mitochondrial disease).[44]

Echocardiography

The diagnosis of HCM relies on the presence of a maximal LV wall thickness of more than 2 standard deviations from the normal (typically $\geq$13 mm in an adult).[1] The hypertrophy is typically asymmetric, involving the interventricular septum more than other segments, but any pattern of LV hypertrophy, including concentric, eccentric, distal, and apical, is consistent with the diagnosis of HCM.[45–48]

In resting conditions, 25% of patients have obstruction to the LV outflow tract.[49,50] As many as 70% of symptomatic patients may have latent, or provokable, LVOTO during maneuvers that increase contractility or reduce afterload and preload. The mechanism of outflow tract obstruction is complex, involving the interaction between the thickened myocardium, the mitral valve leaflets, submitral structures, and altered flow dynamics within the ventricle. In most cases, obstruction is associated with systolic anterior motion (SAM) of the mitral valve, in which the anterior mitral valve leaflet and/or its subvalvular apparatus moves toward and makes contact with the ventricular septum in systole (**Fig. 1**). The most commonly accepted explanation for SAM is that septal hypertrophy, and consequent outflow tract narrowing, produce a high-velocity stream above the mitral valve that causes the tip of the anterior mitral valve leaflet to be sucked against the septum by the Venturi effect. More recent experimental and observational data suggest that abnormalities of the subvalvular apparatus, such as anterior papillary muscle displacement, and primary mitral valve abnormalities, such as accessory mitral tissue,

create leaflet slack to allow SAM at low flows. In this model, the leaflet is driven into the septum like a sail in the wind.[51] Most patients with SAM of the mitral valve have a posteriorly directed jet of mitral regurgitation, but the presence of complex mitral regurgitant jets (eg, anteriorly directed or central) suggests additional abnormalities of the mitral valve. Systolic obliteration of the ventricular cavity can also produce a high-velocity gradient in the midventricle and right ventricular outflow tract obstruction is common in Noonan syndrome and some metabolic disorders.

LV systolic function, assessed from changes in ventricular volume during the cardiac cycle, is typically increased, but regional and long-axis function is usually reduced.[52] A proportion of adults with HCM develop progressive myocardial thinning, global LV systolic impairment, and cavity dilatation.[8] Characteristically, patients with HCM have diastolic LV impairment shown by reduced early diastolic (Ea) velocities in the mitral annulus and septum and reversal of the ratio of early/late diastolic velocities (Ea/Aa).

Cardiac Magnetic Resonance Imaging

Cardiac magnetic resonance imaging provides a detailed assessment of cardiac morphology as well as accurate assessment of systolic function. It also permits tissue characterization, particularly detection of myocardial scarring by the assessment of delayed gadolinium enhancement. Many patients with HCM have areas of patchy gadolinium hyperenhancement, and studies suggest that the extent of gadolinium enhancement correlates with risk factors for sudden death and with progressive LV remodeling.[53–55]

Cardiac Catheterization

Left and right heart catheterization is rarely necessary to make a diagnosis of HCM. The main indications are exclusion of coronary artery disease and, much less commonly, assessment of cardiac output, filling pressures, and intraventricular pressure gradients in patients with severe symptoms. Endomyocardial biopsy is occasionally indicated when an infiltrative or metabolic disease, such as amyloidosis or Anderson-Fabry disease, is suspected.

Exercise Testing

Upright, symptom limited exercise testing is safe in HCM and provides a quantitative assessment of a patient's exercise tolerance, particularly when combined with metabolic functional testing. Patients who do not report symptoms are often found to have suboptimal tests when objectively

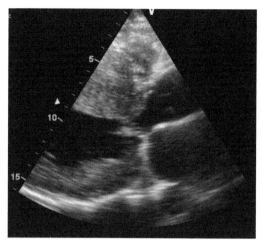

Fig. 1. Systolic Anterior Motion (SAM) of the mitral valve. LVOTO is caused by the anterior leaflet making contact with the septum in systole.

measured. Individuals with HCM usually have a reduced peak oxygen consumption compared with healthy, age-matched controls.[56,57] Twenty-five percent of adults with HCM have an abnormal blood pressure response to exercise, with the blood pressure decreasing or failing to increase by more than 25 mm Hg from baseline.[58,59] This results from abnormal vasodilatation of nonexercising vascular beds triggered by inappropriate firing of LV baroreceptors,[40] and abnormal cardiac output responses.[60] An abnormal blood pressure response to exercise is associated with an increased risk of sudden death in young adults.[59,61]

Ambulatory ECG Monitoring

Ambulatory electrocardiographic monitoring is important in the assessment of symptoms and in the prediction of arrhythmic risk. Nonsustained ventricular tachycardia occurs in 20% of adults with HCM.[62] Most episodes are slow, asymptomatic, and occur during periods of increased vagal tone. In contrast, sustained ventricular tachycardia is uncommon, and may occur in association with apical aneurysms.[63] Paroxysmal supraventricular arrhythmias occur in 30% to 50% of patients; sustained atrial fibrillation (AF) is present in 5% of patients at diagnosis, and develops in a further 10% in the subsequent 5 years.[64,65]

NATURAL HISTORY

HCM can present at any age.[66] Many patients follow a stable and benign course, with a low risk of adverse events, but a minority experience progressive symptoms caused by slow deterioration in LV systolic and diastolic function. A proportion of individuals die suddenly, whereas others may die from progressive heart failure, thromboembolism, and, rarely, infective endocarditis.

Sudden Cardiac Death

HCM is one of the commonest causes of sudden cardiac death in the young. Most contemporary studies report an annual incidence of sudden death in HCM populations of 0.5% to 1% per year, rising to 2% or higher in certain groups.[61–71] The mechanism of sudden cardiac death is rarely documented but factors that contribute to a propensity to ventricular arrhythmia include dispersion of repolarization, which increases susceptibility to triggered arrhythmias; myocyte disarray and areas of conduction block that predispose to reentry arrhythmias; and abnormal ion fluxes during repolarization of myocyte cell membranes causing afterdepolarization and triggered activity. Other morphologic and physiologic factors may influence the vulnerability of the underlying substrate, such as myocardial ischemia, LVOTO, and diastolic dysfunction.

Heart Failure

End-stage HCM develops at all ages but, in most patients, the time from onset of heart failure symptoms to diagnosis of severe systolic impairment is about 10 to 15 years.[8] The development of severe systolic heart failure is associated with a poor prognosis, with rapid progression to death or transplantation and an overall mortality of up to 11% per year.[8] The prevalence of severe systolic impairment in HCM using conventional echocardiographic criteria ranges from 2% to nearly 10%, with an annual incidence of less than 1%.[8,72] However, the true incidence of systolic LV impairment may be much higher because clinically significant reductions in systolic performance may occur while the measured ejection fraction remains within the normal range.

Stroke

The annual incidence of stroke varies from 0.56% to 0.8%/y, rising to 1.9% in patients more than 60 years old.[73] The major cause is atrial fibrillation, which affects about a quarter of patients with HCM, with an incidence of 2% per annum.[64] The odds ratio for stroke in patients with AF is 17.7 (95% confidence interval [CI], 4.1–75.9; P = .0001); 23% of strokes are fatal.[73] Risk factors for AF include age and left atrial dilation (a consequence of diastolic dysfunction, LVOTO, and mitral regurgitation).[64]

Infective Endocarditis

Patients with obstructive HCM have an increased risk of developing infective endocarditis, usually on the anterior mitral valve leaflet.[74] The incidence of infective endocarditis is 1.4 per 1000 person-years (95% CI, 0.5–3.2; 3.8 per 1000 person-years, 95% CI 1.6–8.9, in patients with obstruction).

CLINICAL MANAGEMENT OF HCM

The treatment of most patients with HCM focuses on the counseling of family members, the management of symptoms, and the prevention of disease-related complications. Exceptions include lysosomal storage diseases, such as Pompe and Anderson-Fabry disease, for which specific therapies are available.

Genetic Counseling and Evaluation of Families

All patients with HCM should be counseled on the implications of their diagnosis for other family members.[7] Analysis of carefully constructed family pedigrees can reassure relatives who are not at risk of inheriting the disease. For those who are at risk, current guidelines recommend screening with a 12-lead ECG and echocardiogram at intervals of 12 to 18 months, usually starting at the age of 12 years, unless there is a family history of premature sudden death, the child is symptomatic or a competitive athlete, or there is a clinical suspicion of LV hypertrophy, until full growth and maturation is achieved.[7] Thereafter, if there are no signs of disease expression, clinical screening should be performed every 5 years, because LV hypertrophy can develop well into adulthood. Modified diagnostic criteria that take into account the high probability that otherwise unexplained ECG and echocardiographic findings in first-degree relatives reflect incomplete disease expression should be used when evaluating other family members (**Table 2**). When genetic testing is available, affected individuals should be counseled on the purpose of the test, the likely mode of inheritance, and the potential hazards and limitations of genetic testing.

Table 2
Screening criteria for HCM in first-degree relatives

	Major Criteria	Minor Criteria
Echocardiography	LV wall thickness >13 mm in the anterior septum or posterior wall or >15 mm in the posterior septum or lateral free wall Severe SAM with septal contact	LV wall thickness >12 mm in the anterior septum or posterior wall or >14 mm in the posterior septum or lateral free wall Moderate SAM with no septal contact Redundant mitral valve leaflets
Electrocardiography	Left ventricular hypertrophy and repolarization changes (Romhilt-Estes) Abnormal Q (>40 ms or >25% R wave) in at least 2 leads from II, III, aVF (in absence of left anterior hemiblock), V1–V4; or I, aVl, V5–V6 T wave inversion in leads I and aVL (>3 mm) (with QRS-T wave axis difference >30°), V3–V6 (>3 mm) or II and III and aVF (>5 mm)	Complete BBB or (minor) interventricular conduction defect (in LV leads) Deep S V2 (>25 mm) Minor repolarization changes in LV leads

Abbreviation: BBB, bundle branch block.

Data from McKenna WJ, Spirito P, Desnos M, et al. Experience from clinical genetics in hypertrophic cardiomyopathy: proposal for new diagnostic criteria in adult members of affected families. Heart 1997;77:131.

Symptom Management

In patients with symptoms caused by LVOTO, the aim of treatment is to reduce the outflow tract gradient. Options include negatively inotropic drugs (β-blockers, disopyramide, and verapamil), atrioventricular sequential pacing, percutaneous alcohol ablation of the interventricular septum, and surgery.

Approximately 60% to 70% of patients improve with medical therapy but high doses are frequently required and side effects are common.[7] Dual-chamber pacing using a short-programmed atrioventricular delay to produce maximum preexcitation while maintaining effective atrial transport can reduce the outflow gradient by 30% to 50%, but provides little objective improvement in exercise capacity in most patients.[75] Selective injection of alcohol into a septal perforator branch of the left anterior descending coronary artery to create a localized septal scar can be effective, but is associated with atrioventricular block requiring a pacemaker in 5% to 20% of patients and is unsuitable for all patients because of variation in coronary artery anatomy and coexistent mitral valve abnormalities.[76]

Surgery is considered in patients with significant outflow obstruction (gradient >50 mm Hg) and symptoms refractory to medical therapy. The most commonly performed surgical procedure, ventricular septal myectomy, substantially reduces the gradient and improves exercise capacity and symptoms. In experienced centers, mortalities are less than 1% and complications such as atrioventricular block and ventricular septal defects are rare.[77]

Therapeutic options in patients without LV outflow gradients are limited predominantly to pharmacologic therapy. β-Blockade, calcium antagonists such as verapamil, and diltiazem can relieve chest pain and dyspnea. In patients with paroxysmal nocturnal dyspnea and chronically raised pulmonary pressures, diuretics can be effective, but the dose and duration of therapy should be minimized, particularly in patients with severe diastolic impairment or labile obstruction. At present, pharmacologic therapy for systolic heart failure in HCM is initiated only when patients develop symptoms and a low ejection fraction. The drugs used (angiotensin-converting enzyme inhibitors or angiotensin receptor blockers, β-adrenoreceptor blockers, diuretics, and digoxin) are identical to those used at an earlier stage in patients with dilated cardiomyopathy. In HCM, the benefit of treatment at this later stage is unknown, but it may not substantially improve prognosis.

Management of Atrial Arrhythmia

Anticoagulation should be considered in all patients with sustained or paroxysmal AF. Treatment with low-dose amiodarone, 1000 to 1400 mg/wk, is effective in maintaining sinus rhythm and in controlling the ventricular response during breakthrough episodes. The addition of a low-dose β-blocker, verapamil, or diltiazem may be required for rate control. In general, the principles of managing AF in patients with HCM are similar to those in other conditions, with the proviso that the threshold to use anticoagulation should be lower.

Prevention of Sudden Cardiac Death

The published annual incidence of sudden cardiac death in patients with HCM has declined from between 2% and 4% to 1% or less.[78,79] The reasons for this change are complex and relate not only to medical intervention but also to the identification of patients with milder disease. Sudden cardiac death occurs throughout life, with a maximum incidence in adolescence and young adulthood, often without warning signs or symptoms.[62] Although there is an excess of deaths during or after strenuous exertion, most occur during mild exertion or sedentary activities.[7] The mechanism underlying most sudden cardiac deaths is believed to be ventricular tachyarrhythmia, but conduction disease and thromboembolism may account for some cases.[7] Rapid AF and myocardial ischemia seem to be important triggers for sudden ventricular arrhythmia.[80]

Although sudden death rates are generally low, sudden death frequently occurs without warning in young and often mildly symptomatic individuals, which is a powerful motive to preemptively identify patients at high risk; however, this is challenging because of the different causes of HCM, a heterogeneous clinical phenotype, and evolution of the arrhythmogenic substrate with time. Nevertheless, it is possible to identify a high-risk cohort using a small number of readily determined clinical parameters (**Table 3**).[7,81] There is general acceptance that the risk associated with individual risk factors is cumulative. The significance of risk factors must also be assessed in relation to age and the presence of modifiers such as LVOTO.

In general, the presence of 2 or more conventional risk factors should prompt consideration of an implantable cardioverter defibrillator (ICD), because patients with 2 or more risk factors have a 4% to 5% annual risk of sudden cardiac death (**Table 4**).[7] More problematic are patients who

Table 3
Clinical parameters associated with sudden cardiac death (SCD)

Major Clinical Parameter	PPV (%)	NPV (%)
Nonsustained ventricular arrhythmia	25	85
Family history of SCD	28	88
Unexplained syncope	25	86
Maximal wall thickness ≥30 mm	13	95
Abnormal blood pressure response to exercise	15	>95

Abbreviations: NPV, negative predictive value; PPV, positive predictive value.

Data from Maron BJ, McKenna WJ, Danielson GK, et al. American College of Cardiology/European Society of Cardiology Clinical Expert Consensus Document on Hypertrophic Cardiomyopathy: a report of the American College of Cardiology Foundation Task Force on Clinical Expert Consensus Documents and the European Society of Cardiology Committee for Practice Guidelines. Eur Heart J 2003;24(21):1980–2; Frenneaux MP. Assessing the risk of sudden cardiac death in a patient with hypertrophic cardiomyopathy. Heart 2004;90(5):572.

have only a single risk factor (up to 25% of patients). When assessing the need for ICDs in this group, age, symptoms, and the presence of so-called minor risk factors should be taken into account and balanced against the risk of complications of ICD therapy, particularly in young people.[81]

Patients with HCM and risk factors should refrain from intense exercise. This restriction has significant implications for many patients, underlining the importance of accurate diagnosis.

Role of Electrophysiologic Testing in HCM

Current guidelines suggest that electrophysiologic testing might have a role in some borderline cases,[82] but 36% of patients have inducible sustained ventricular tachycardia when protocols consisting of 3 premature stimuli delivered during 3 drive pacing cycle lengths in the left and/or right ventricle are used.[83] Ventricular tachycardia induced by such aggressive protocols may be associated with a higher risk of cardiac events but, because the predictive accuracy for sudden death is low, routine use of electrophysiology testing is not recommended.[83] One study has suggested that paced ventricular electrogram fractionation may have greater value for predicting sudden cardiac death than conventional invasive criteria or the noninvasive risk factors, but the exact role of this technique requires evaluation in larger populations.[84]

Pregnancy

Serious complications during pregnancy in women with HCM occur in less than 2% of pregnancies. Maternal mortality seems to be confined to women

Table 4
ACC/AHA/ESC guidelines for ICD prescription in HCM

Guideline	Indication Class	Level of Evidence
ICD therapy should be used for treatment in patients with HCM who have sustained ventricular tachycardia and/or ventricular fibrillation	I	B
ICD implantation can be effective for primary prophylaxis against SCD in patients with HCM who have 1 or more major risk factor (see **Table 3**) for SCD	IIa	C
Electrophysiologic testing may be considered for risk assessment for SCD in patients with HCM	IIb	C

The classes of ICD indications as defined by the ACC/AHA/ESC Writing Committee are summarized. They refer to individuals who are receiving chronic optimal medical therapy and otherwise have reasonable expectation of survival with a good functional status for more than 1 year.

Data from Zipes DP, Camm AJ, Borggrefe M, et al. ACC/AHA/ESC 2006 Guidelines for management of patients with ventricular arrhythmias and the prevention of sudden cardiac death: a report of the American College of Cardiology/American Heart Association Task Force and the European Society of Cardiology Committee for Practice Guidelines (Writing Committee to Develop Guidelines for Management of Patients With Ventricular Arrhythmias and the Prevention of Sudden Cardiac Death). J Am Coll Cardiol 2006;48(5):e293.

with high risk profiles.[85,86] The vasodilation associated with standard epidural analgesia may worsen LVOTO, and care must be taken when administering cardioactive drugs. In general, most pregnant women with HCM undergo normal vaginal delivery without the need for cesarean section; all should be offered specialized obstetric antenatal and perinatal care.

REFERENCES

1. Elliott P, Andersson B, Arbustini E, et al. Classification of the cardiomyopathies: a position statement from the European Society of Cardiology Working Group on Myocardial and Pericardial Diseases. Eur Heart J 2008;29(2):270–6.
2. Maron BJ, Gardin JM, Flack JM, et al. Prevalence of hypertrophic cardiomyopathy in a general population of young adults. Echocardiographic analysis of 4111 subjects in the CARDIA Study. Coronary Artery Risk Development in (Young) Adults. Circulation 1995;92(4):785–9.
3. Marian AJ, Roberts R. The molecular genetic basis for hypertrophic cardiomyopathy. J Mol Cell Cardiol 2001;33(4):655–70.
4. Richard P, Charron P, Carrier L, et al. Hypertrophic cardiomyopathy: distribution of disease genes, spectrum of mutations, and implications for a molecular diagnosis strategy. EUROGENE heart failure project. Circulation 2003;107(17):2227–32.
5. Seidman JG, Seidman C. The genetic basis for cardiomyopathy: from mutation identification to mechanistic paradigms. Cell 2001;104(4):557–67.
6. Maron BJ, Estes NA 3rd, Maron MS, et al. Primary prevention of sudden death as a novel treatment strategy in hypertrophic cardiomyopathy. Circulation 2003;107(23):2872–5.
7. Maron BJ, McKenna WJ, Danielson GK, et al. Task force on clinical expert consensus documents. American College of Cardiology; Committee for Practice Guidelines. European Society of Cardiology. J Am Coll Cardiol 2003;42(9):1687–713.
8. Thaman R, Gimeno JR, Murphy RT, et al. Prevalence and clinical significance of systolic impairment in hypertrophic cardiomyopathy. Heart 2005;91(7):920–5.
9. Kubo T, Gimeno JR, Bahl A, et al. Prevalence, clinical significance, and genetic basis of hypertrophic cardiomyopathy with restrictive phenotype. J Am Coll Cardiol 2007;49(25):2419–26.
10. Alcalai R, Seidman JG, Seidman CE. Genetic basis of hypertrophic cardiomyopathy: from bench to the clinics. J Cardiovasc Electrophysiol 2008;19(1):104–10.
11. Perkins MJ, Van Driest SL, Ellsworth EG. Gene-specific modifying effects of pro-LVH polymorphisms involving the renin-angiotensin-aldosterone system among 389 unrelated patients with hypertrophic cardiomyopathy. Eur Heart J 2005;26(22):2457–62.
12. Lind JM, Chiu C, Ingles J, et al. Sex hormone receptor gene variation associated with phenotype in male hypertrophic cardiomyopathy patients. J Mol Cell Cardiol 2008;45(2):217–22.
13. Nagai T, Ogimoto A, Okayama H, et al. A985G polymorphism of the endothelin-2 gene and atrial fibrillation in patients with hypertrophic cardiomyopathy. Circ J 2007;71(12):1932–6.
14. Tartaglia M, Gelb BD. Noonan syndrome and related disorders: genetics and pathogenesis. Annu Rev Genomics Hum Genet 2005;6:45–68.
15. Noonan JA. Hypertelorism with Turner phenotype. A new syndrome with associated congenital heart disease. Am J Dis Child 1968;116(4):373–80.
16. Sharland M, Burch M, McKenna WM, et al. A clinical study of Noonan syndrome. Arch Dis Child 1992;67(2):178–83.
17. Tartaglia M, Mehler EL, Goldberg R, et al. Mutations in PTPN11, encoding the protein tyrosine phosphatase SHP-2, cause Noonan syndrome. Nat Genet 2001;29(4):465–8.
18. Tartaglia M, Pennacchio LA, Zhao C, et al. Gain-of-function SOS1 mutations cause a distinctive form of Noonan syndrome. Nat Genet 2007;39(1):75–9.
19. Roberts AE, Araki T, Swanson KD, et al. Germline gain-of-function mutations in SOS1 cause Noonan syndrome. Nat Genet 2007;39(1):70–4.
20. Schubbert S, Zenker M, Rowe SL, et al. Germline KRAS mutations cause Noonan syndrome. Nat Genet 2006;38(3):331–6.
21. Pandit B, Sarkozy A, Pennacchio LA, et al. Gain-of-function RAF1 mutations cause Noonan and LEOPARD syndromes with hypertrophic cardiomyopathy. Nat Genet 2007;39(8):1007–12.
22. Razzaque MA, Nishizawa T, Komoike Y, et al. Germline gain-of-function mutations in RAF1 cause Noonan syndrome. Nat Genet 2007;39(8):1013–7.
23. Digilio MC, Conti E, Sarkozy A, et al. Grouping of multiple-lentigines/LEOPARD and Noonan syndromes on the PTPN11 gene. Am J Hum Genet 2002;71(2):389–94.
24. Linhart A, Elliott PM. The heart in Anderson-Fabry disease and other lysosomal storage disorders. Heart 2007;93(4):528–35.
25. Nishino I, Fu J, Tanji K, et al. Primary LAMP-2 deficiency causes X-linked vacuolar cardiomyopathy and myopathy (Danon disease). Nature 2000;406(6798):906–10.
26. Danon MJ, Oh SJ, DiMauro S, et al. Lysosomal glycogen storage disease with normal acid maltase. Neurology 1981;31(1):51–7.
27. Sugie K, Yamamoto A, Murayama K, et al. Clinico-pathological features of genetically confirmed Danon disease. Neurology 2002;58(12):1773–8.

28. Katzin LW, Amato AA. Pompe disease: a review of the current diagnosis and treatment recommendations in the era of enzyme replacement therapy. J Clin Neuromuscul Dis 2008;9(4):421–31.

29. Klinge L, Straub V, Neudorf U, et al. Enzyme replacement therapy in classical infantile Pompe disease: results of a ten-month follow-up study. Neuropediatrics 2005;36(1):6–11.

30. Blair E, Redwood C, Ashrafian H, et al. Mutations in the gamma(2) subunit of AMP-activated protein kinase cause familial hypertrophic cardiomyopathy: evidence for the central role of energy compromise in disease pathogenesis. Hum Mol Genet 2001; 10(11):1215–20.

31. Murphy RT, Mogensen J, McGarry K, et al. Adenosine monophosphate-activated protein kinase disease mimics hypertrophic cardiomyopathy and Wolff-Parkinson-White syndrome: natural history. J Am Coll Cardiol 2005;45(6):922–30.

32. Scaglia F, Towbin JA, Craigen WJ, et al. Clinical spectrum, morbidity, and mortality in 113 pediatric patients with mitochondrial disease. Pediatrics 2004;114(4):925–31.

33. Holmgren D, Wåhlander H, Eriksson BO, et al. Cardiomyopathy in children with mitochondrial disease; clinical course and cardiological findings. Eur Heart J 2003;24(3):280–8.

34. Alper G, Narayanan V. Friedreich's ataxia. Pediatr Neurol 2003;28(5):335–41.

35. Child JS, Perloff JK, Bach PM, et al. Cardiac involvement in Friedreich's ataxia: a clinical study of 75 patients. J Am Coll Cardiol 1986;7(6):1370–8.

36. Casazza F, Ferrari F, Piccone U, et al. Progression of cardiopathology in Friedreich ataxia: clinico-instrumental study. Cardiologia 1990;35(5):423–31.

37. Davies MJ, McKenna WJ. Hypertrophic cardiomyopathy—pathology and pathogenesis. Histopathology 1995;26(6):493–500.

38. Hughes SE. The pathology of hypertrophic cardiomyopathy. Histopathology 2004;44(5):412–27.

39. Maron BJ, Wolfson JK, Epstein SE, et al. Intramural ("small vessel") coronary artery disease in hypertrophic cardiomyopathy. J Am Coll Cardiol 1986;8(3): 545–57.

40. Counihan PJ, Frenneaux MP, Webb DJ, et al. Abnormal vascular responses to supine exercise in hypertrophic cardiomyopathy. Circulation 1991; 84(2):686–96.

41. Elliott P, McKenna WJ. Hypertrophic cardiomyopathy. Lancet 2004;363(9424):1881–91.

42. Yamaguchi H, Ishimura T, Nishiyama S, et al. Hypertrophic nonobstructive cardiomyopathy with giant negative T waves (apical hypertrophy): ventriculographic and echocardiographic features in 30 patients. Am J Cardiol 1979;44(3):401–12.

43. Fananapazir L, Tracy CM, Leon MB, et al. Electrophysiologic abnormalities in patients with hypertrophic cardiomyopathy. A consecutive analysis in 155 patients. Circulation 1989;80(5):1259–68.

44. Krikler DM, Davies MJ, Rowland E, et al. Sudden death in hypertrophic cardiomyopathy: associated accessory atrioventricular pathways. Br Heart J 1980;43(3):245–51.

45. Klues HG, Schiffers A, Maron BJ. Phenotypic spectrum and patterns of left ventricular hypertrophy in hypertrophic cardiomyopathy: morphologic observations and significance as assessed by two-dimensional echocardiography in 600 patients. J Am Coll Cardiol 1995;26(7):1699–708.

46. Maron BJ, Gottdiener JS, Epstein SE. Patterns and significance of distribution of left ventricular hypertrophy in hypertrophic cardiomyopathy. A wide angle, two dimensional echocardiographic study of 125 patients. Am J Cardiol 1981;48(3):418–28.

47. Shapiro LM, McKenna WJ. Distribution of left ventricular hypertrophy in hypertrophic cardiomyopathy: a two-dimensional echocardiographic study. J Am Coll Cardiol 1983;2(3):437–44.

48. Wigle ED, Sasson Z, Henderson MA, et al. Hypertrophic cardiomyopathy. The importance of the site and the extent of hypertrophy [a review]. Prog Cardiovasc Dis 1985;28(1):1–83.

49. Maron MS, Olivotto I, Zenovich AG, et al. Hypertrophic cardiomyopathy is predominantly a disease of left ventricular outflow tract obstruction. Circulation 2006;114(21):2232–9.

50. Shah JS, Esteban MT, Thaman R, et al. Prevalence of exercise-induced left ventricular outflow tract obstruction in symptomatic patients with non-obstructive hypertrophic cardiomyopathy. Heart 2008;94(10):1288–94.

51. Robert A, Levine MD, Gus J, et al. Papillary muscle displacement causes systolic anterior motion of the mitral valve; experimental validation and insights into the mechanism of subaortic obstruction. Circulation 1995;91:1189–95.

52. Kramer CM, Reichek N, Ferrari VA, et al. Regional heterogeneity of function in hypertrophic cardiomyopathy. Circulation 1994;90(1):186–94.

53. Choudhury L, Mahrholdt H, Wagner A, et al. Myocardial scarring in asymptomatic or mildly symptomatic patients with hypertrophic cardiomyopathy. J Am Coll Cardiol 2002;40(12):2156–64.

54. Moon JC, McKenna WJ, McCrohon JA, et al. Toward clinical risk assessment in hypertrophic cardiomyopathy with gadolinium cardiovascular magnetic resonance. J Am Coll Cardiol 2003;41(9):1561–7.

55. O'Hanlon R, Grasso A, Roughton M, et al. Prognostic significance of myocardial fibrosis in hypertrophic cardiomyopathy. J Am Coll Cardiol 2010; 56(11):867–74.

56. Jones S, Elliott PM, Sharma S, et al. Cardiopulmonary responses to exercise in patients with hypertrophic cardiomyopathy. Heart 1998;80(1):60–7.

57. Sharma S, Elliott PM, Whyte G, et al. Utility of metabolic exercise testing in distinguishing hypertrophic cardiomyopathy from physiologic left ventricular hypertrophy in athletes. J Am Coll Cardiol 2000; 36(3):864–70.

58. Olivotto I, Maron BJ, Montereggi A, et al. Prognostic value of systemic blood pressure response during exercise in a community-based patient population with hypertrophic cardiomyopathy. J Am Coll Cardiol 1999;33(7):2044–51.

59. Sadoul N, Prasad K, Elliott PM, et al. Prospective prognostic assessment of blood pressure response during exercise in patients with hypertrophic cardiomyopathy. Circulation 1997;96(9):2987–91.

60. Ciampi Q, Betocchi S, Lombardi R, et al. Hemodynamic determinants of exercise-induced abnormal blood pressure response in hypertrophic cardiomyopathy. J Am Coll Cardiol 2002;40(2):278–84.

61. Elliott PM, Poloniecki J, Dickie S, et al. Sudden death in hypertrophic cardiomyopathy: identification of high risk patients. J Am Coll Cardiol 2000;36(7): 2212–8.

62. Monserrat L, Elliott PM, Gimeno JR, et al. Non-sustained ventricular tachycardia in hypertrophic cardiomyopathy: an independent marker of sudden death risk in young patients. J Am Coll Cardiol 2003; 42(5):873–9.

63. Sanghvi NK, Tracy CM. Sustained ventricular tachycardia in apical hypertrophic cardiomyopathy, mid-cavitary obstruction, and apical aneurysm. Pacing Clin Electrophysiol 2007;30(6):799–803.

64. Olivotto I, Cecchi F, Casey SA, et al. Impact of atrial fibrillation on the clinical course of hypertrophic cardiomyopathy. Circulation 2001;104(21): 2517–24.

65. Robinson K, Frenneaux MP, Stockins B, et al. Atrial fibrillation in hypertrophic cardiomyopathy: a longitudinal study. J Am Coll Cardiol 1990;15(6):1279–85.

66. Maron BJ, Casey SA, Hauser RG, et al. Clinical course of hypertrophic cardiomyopathy with survival to advanced age. J Am Coll Cardiol 2003;42(5): 882–8.

67. Maron BJ, Spirito P. Impact of patient selection biases on the perception of hypertrophic cardiomyopathy and its natural history. Am J Cardiol 1993; 72(12):970–2.

68. Colan SD, Lipshultz SE, Lowe AM, et al. Epidemiology and cause-specific outcome of hypertrophic cardiomyopathy in children: findings from the Pediatric Cardiomyopathy Registry. Circulation 2007; 115(6):773–81.

69. Maron BJ. Hypertrophic cardiomyopathy in childhood. Pediatr Clin North Am 2004;51(5):1305–46.

70. Spirito P, Chiarella F, Carratino L, et al. Clinical course and prognosis of hypertrophic cardiomyopathy in an outpatient population. N Engl J Med 1989;320(12): 749–55.

71. Spirito P, Rapezzi C, Autore C, et al. Prognosis of asymptomatic patients with hypertrophic cardiomyopathy and nonsustained ventricular tachycardia. Circulation 1994;90(6):2743–7.

72. Spirito P, Maron BJ, Bonow RO, et al. Occurrence and significance of progressive left ventricular wall thinning and relative cavity dilatation in patients with hypertrophic cardiomyopathy. Am J Cardiol 1987;60:123–9.

73. Maron BJ, Olivotto I, Bellone P, et al. Clinical profile of stroke in 900 patients with hypertrophic cardiomyopathy. J Am Coll Cardiol 2002;39(2):301–7.

74. Spirito P, Rapezzi C, Bellone P, et al. Infective endocarditis in hypertrophic cardiomyopathy: prevalence, incidence, and indications for antibiotic prophylaxis. Circulation 1999;99(16):2132–7.

75. Maron BJ, Nishimura RA, McKenna WJ, et al. Assessment of permanent dual-chamber pacing as a treatment for drug-refractory symptomatic patients with obstructive hypertrophic cardiomyopathy. A randomized, double-blind, crossover study (M-PATHY). Circulation 1999;99(22):2927–33.

76. Maron BJ. Role of alcohol septal ablation in treatment of obstructive hypertrophic cardiomyopathy. Lancet 2000;355(9202):425–6.

77. Merrill WH, Friesinger GC, Graham TP Jr, et al. Long-lasting improvement after septal myectomy for hypertrophic obstructive cardiomyopathy. Ann Thorac Surg 2000;69(6):1732–5 [discussion: 1735–6].

78. Maron BJ, Shirani J, Poliac LC, et al. Sudden death in young competitive athletes. Clinical, demographic, and pathological profiles. JAMA 1996; 276(3):199–204.

79. Elliott PM, Sharma S, Varnava A, et al. Survival after cardiac arrest or sustained ventricular tachycardia in patients with hypertrophic cardiomyopathy. J Am Coll Cardiol 1999;33(6):1596–601.

80. Dilsizian V, Bonow RO, Epstein SE, et al. Myocardial ischemia detected by thallium scintigraphy is frequently related to cardiac arrest and syncope in young patients with hypertrophic cardiomyopathy. J Am Coll Cardiol 1993;22(3):796–804.

81. Frenneaux MP. Assessing the risk of sudden cardiac death in a patient with hypertrophic cardiomyopathy. Heart 2004;90(5):570–5.

82. Garratt CJ, Elliott P, Behr E, et al. Heart rhythm UK Familial Sudden Cardiac Death Syndromes Statement Development Group. Heart rhythm UK position statement on clinical indications for implantable cardioverter defibrillators in adult patients with familial sudden cardiac death syndromes. Europace 2010; 12(8):1156–75.

83. Behr ER, Elliott P, McKenna WJ. Role of invasive EP testing in the evaluation and management of hypertrophic cardiomyopathy. Card Electrophysiol Rev 2002;6(4):482–6.

84. Saumarez RC, Pytkowski M, Sterlinski M, et al. Paced ventricular electrogram fractionation predicts sudden cardiac death in hypertrophic cardiomyopathy. Eur Heart J 2008;29(13):1653–61.

85. Autore C, Conte MR, Piccininno M, et al. Risk associated with pregnancy in hypertrophic cardiomyopathy. J Am Coll Cardiol 2002;40(10): 1864–9.

86. Thaman R, Varnava A, Hamid MS, et al. Pregnancy related complications in women with hypertrophic cardiomyopathy. Heart 2003;89(7): 752–6.

Genetics of Dilated Cardiomyopathy: Risk of Conduction Defects and Sudden Cardiac Death

Samer Arnous, MBBS, MRCPI[a], Petros Syrris, PhD[b],
Srijita Sen-Chowdhry, MRCP, MD, FESC[b,c],
William J. McKenna, MD, DSc, FRCP, FESC[a,b],*

KEYWORDS

- Arrhythmia • Familial dilated cardiomyopathy
- Sudden cardiac death • Conduction defect • Laminopathy
- Left ventricular arrhythmogenic cardiomyopathy

Dilated cardiomyopathy (DCM) is a chronic progressive myocardial disorder with an annual incidence of 6 to 8 cases/100,000 population and prevalence of 36.5 cases/100,000 population.[1] It remains a leading cause of heart failure in people younger than 35 years and the most common indication for cardiac transplantation worldwide.[2,3] The reported frequencies probably represent an underestimate, however, because most studies focus on index cases presenting with clinical heart failure. Recognition of the familial and genetic basis of DCM is relatively recent.

In index cases, DCM is diagnosed in the presence of depressed fractional shortening (<25%) or reduced left ventricular ejection fraction (LVEF) (<45%), and a dilated left ventricle (end-diastolic diameter >117% of the predicted value corrected for age and body surface area).[4] Incomplete phenotypic expression is common among relatives, contributing to underrecognition of familial disease. Nevertheless, nearly a third of asymptomatic relatives of patients with DCM have echocardiographic abnormalities on screening (eg, depressed fractional shortening, left ventricular enlargement), and more than a quarter of these patients develop overt DCM.[5] Furthermore, cardiac-specific autoantibodies were present in more than 30% of asymptomatic relatives of patients with DCM,[6,7] and are weak independent predictors of DCM development at 5-year follow-up.[7,8]

In a longitudinal study of families with DCM, 23% of 767 asymptomatic relatives were found to have echocardiographic evidence of depressed fractional shortening or left ventricular dilation, and these patients were eight times more likely to develop overt DCM than those with normal echocardiograms.[9] Additional studies in the asymptomatic relatives showed that the 25% of relatives with left ventricular enlargement (LVE) without systolic dysfunction had histologic findings consistent with DCM,[10] significant reduction

This work was undertaken at UCLH/UCL, which received a proportion of funding from the Department of Health's NIHR Biomedical Research Centres funding scheme.
The authors have nothing to disclose.
[a] Inherited Cardiovascular Disease Group, University College London Hospitals NHS Trust, The Heart Hospital, 16-18 Westmoreland Street, Westminster, London W1G 8PH, UK
[b] Inherited Cardiovascular Disease Group, Institute of Cardiovascular Science, University College London, Paul O'Gorman Building, 72 Huntley Street, Camden, London WC1E 6DD, UK
[c] Department of Epidemiology, Imperial College- St Mary's Campus, Norfolk Place, London W2 1NY, UK
* Corresponding author. Inherited Cardiovascular Disease Group, University College London Hospitals NHS Trust, The Heart Hospital, 16-18 Westmoreland Street, Westminster, London W1G 8PH, UK.
E-mail address: william.mckenna@uclh.org

in exercise capacity,[5,11] and a prolonged QRS complex on signal-averaged ECG, in contrast to normal relatives.[5] This finding suggests that LVE represents subclinical disease, with incomplete phenotypic expression. Despite reduced penetrance, variable expressivity, and the small nuclear families commonly evaluated in clinical practice, familial disease can be confirmed in up to 50% of DCM cases. Familial DCM is diagnosed in the presence of at least two affected individuals in the same family, or a history of unexplained sudden cardiac death (SCD) before the age of 35 years in a first-degree relative.

The prognosis of DCM is highly variable. Earlier studies reported 5-year mortality rates of 50%, which have declined to 20% in more recent reports. This improvement in survival reflects both advances in heart failure therapy and early disease detection. Previously, most patients in any DCM cohort presented with symptoms of high pulmonary venous pressure and a low cardiac output. Increasingly, DCM is diagnosed as an incidental finding in asymptomatic individuals during routine examination or family screening.[5,12,13]

Currently patients with DCM are treated according to international guidelines for the management of heart failure, which are backed by clinical trials. However, a significant knowledge gap remains. The optimal approach to forestalling progression in relatives with early disease is unresolved. Furthermore, there is an unmet need to individualize standard therapies, which do not factor in the influence of underlying cause on treatment responsiveness. Recent studies suggest that this might result in suboptimal or inappropriate therapy in some patients.[14–16] The influence of genetic factors in determining the response (and timing) of drug therapy is largely unstudied in DCM. Heterogeneity in age of onset, clinical manifestations, and outcome is observed within families, implying that factors other than the primary mutation influence phenotype and prognosis.

An important unsolved challenge in the management of DCM is individual assessment of the lifetime risk of SCD. Scant data exist on the natural history associated with specific genetic mutations and predisposition to arrhythmia. However, recent studies have shown that the arrhythmogenic risk is higher in certain subtypes of DCM, such as the laminopathies.

This article focuses on the heterogeneity of phenotypic expression in familial DCM, with emphasis on the various gene mutations associated with increased risk of high-grade atrioventricular block, malignant ventricular arrhythmias, and SCD.

GENETICS

More than 40 disease-causing genes have been identified in DCM,[17] most of which encode proteins of the sarcolemma,[18–20] cytoskeleton,[21] sarcomere,[22–26] nuclear envelope (eg, Lamin[27–29]), and mitochondrion[30] (**Table 1**). The structural and functional consequences DCM mutations include impairment of myocardial force generation, force transmission, and cell survival (**Fig. 1**).

DCM is inherited as an autosomal dominant trait in 90% of families. This mode of transmission is often associated with reduced and age-related penetrance (**Table 2**), although onset by the fourth decade of life is typical.[13] Expression is also variable and frequently incomplete; although symptomatic disease may not be present, cardiac evaluation may reveal unexplained electrocardiogram (ECG) or echocardiographic abnormalities. Autosomal dominant forms of DCM may be associated with conduction disease[76] or skeletal myopathy.[52,77]

Other modes of inheritance include autosomal recessive, X-linked recessive, and mitochondrial. In autosomal recessive DCM, patients usually present at a younger age than those with the dominant form. The disease course is characterized by more rapid progression to death or cardiac transplantation.[13] X-linked inheritance is characterized by the absence of male-to-male transmission.[13,78] Women may be affected but usually express a milder form of disease expression with onset later in life. Affected patients usually have an increase in creatine kinase (CK)-MM isoform level (eg, mutations in dystrophin that also cause Duchenne and Becker muscular dystrophy).

Matrilineal inheritance is usually associated with signs of mitochondrial-related phenotype, such as lactacidemia, hypoacusia, palpebral ptosis, myopathy with ragged red fibers, ophthalmoplegia, encephalopathy, or retinitis pigmentosa. In this form of inheritance the mother, son, or daughter may be affected, but the affected men do not transmit the disease to their offspring.

DCM WITH ARRHYTHMIA AS INITIAL PRESENTATION
Laminopathies

A large number of mutations have been identified in LMNA, the gene encoding lamins A and C, which is 12 exons in length and located on the long arm of chromosome 1 (1q21.2-q21.3). Phenotypic manifestations are diverse, including an array of rare but dominantly transmitted diseases affecting cardiac and skeletal muscle (laminopathies): Emery-Dreifuss muscular dystrophy,[29,79]

Dunnigan-type familial partial lipodystrophy (a rare degenerative disorder of the adipose tissue),[80,81] limb girdle muscular dystrophy 1B,[82] and dilated cardiomyopathy with conduction system disease.[27,52,53] Although initial reports have emphasized that patients with DCM from lamin A/C (LMNA) mutation often have a conduction defect or atrial fibrillation before the development of heart failure, it is increasingly apparent that SCD from ventricular arrhythmia is a major prognostic determinant, and often occurs before the onset of severe left ventricular dysfunction.[83]

The marked phenotypic heterogeneity observed in conjunction with LMNA mutations may be related to the myriad functional roles of the protein product. The nuclear envelope separates the nucleus from the cytoplasm and provides it with mechanical support. Integral to it is the nuclear lamina, a network of intermediate filaments composed of type A and B lamin proteins. Lamin A and C are the most common A-type lamins. While B-type lamins are expressed in all tissue and cell types, A-type lamins are expressed only in terminally differentiated tissue, such as skeletal and cardiac muscle,[84] and therefore mutations in LMNA will primarily affect these tissues. Lamins not only provide structural scaffolding for the cell nucleus[85] but also are involved in regulating DNA replication and transcription,[86] cell cycle regulation, cell differentiation, and apoptosis. Therefore, lamin mutations may cause disruption of nuclear function, resulting in cell death. Mice lacking the LMNA gene have been shown to develop rapidly progressive DCM with conduction defects (slow heart rates, prolonged PR and QRS intervals).[87]

LMNA gene mutations were first described by Bonne and colleagues[29] in a large French family with autosomal dominant Emery-Dreifuss muscular dystrophy, a genetic disorder characterized by early-onset contractures, progressive muscular wasting and weakness with humeroperoneal distribution, and cardiac conduction defects. Of the affected individuals with LMNA mutations, 70% presented with isolated cardiac involvement characterized by severe atrioventricular conduction defects and sinus node dysfunction.[88] Of the 15 deceased individuals, 8 had suffered SCD, despite prior implantation of a pacemaker in 3. The first cardiac symptoms were marked atrioventricular conduction defects or sinus dysfunction, with a rapid progression to ventricular dysfunction and severe DCM. The mean age of onset of cardiac symptoms was 33 years.

Current data support the view that LMNA mutations are among the most common defects in familial DCM, accounting for 5–8% of all DCM cases,[27,28,54−57] and up to 70% of cases of DCM with conduction defects and/or muscle contractures.[54]

Novel mutations in LMNA were also identified in a family with a high incidence of asymptomatic conduction defects in the third and fourth decades, which progressed to high grade atrioventricular block requiring permanent pacemaker insertion. DCM developed in the fifth and sixth decades, indicating that conduction defects may precede the development of DCM in LMNA disease.[53]

Atrial flutter/fibrillation is a prominent feature in some kindreds. Fatkin and colleagues reported on families carrying the N195K and L85R mutations in LMNA; the prevalence of atrial fibrillation was 91 and 100%, while DCM was present in 73% and 100%, respectively. Conduction system disease was common in both families.[27] In another family with an E161K mutation in LMNA, all five adults carrying the mutation had atrial fibrillation, but only two had DCM; therefore atrial fibrillation was the first symptom of the disease in these cases.[57] This finding is in contrast with the usual proposed natural history of DCM, in which atrial fibrillation usually follows the development of impaired left ventricular function.

In contrast to other DCM patients, symptomatic LMNA carriers appear to have significantly higher mortality from SCD and heart failure.[28,55] Clinical predictors of carrier status include the presence of supraventricular arrhythmia, conduction disease, and skeletal muscle involvement. A trend towards younger age of clinical onset (mean 27 years) has also been reported. Carriers had a lesser degree of left ventricular dilation after correction for body surface area and age (mean left ventricular diastolic diameter for carriers vs noncarrier DCM patients was 5.02 and 6.41 cm, respectively). By the age of 45 years, the risk of cardiovascular death and cardiac transplant were significantly higher in the LMNA mutation carriers. Of 12 carriers of LMNA mutations, 8 were deceased, required heart transplantation, or had severe worsening of myocardial function between the third and fifth decade.

In a meta-analysis of nearly 300 carriers of a LMNA mutation, 92% of those older than 30 years had conduction defects, with 44% requiring permanent pacemaker implantation.[16] The most characteristic finding on resting ECG was the presence of low amplitude P wave, first-degree atrioventricular block, and normal QRS width. Among patients with LMNA mutations, 46% of deaths were sudden, whereas 12% were from heart failure. The risk of SCD was significantly increased compared with the normal population or carriers of sarcomeric mutations.[16] Although a high

Table 1
Gene mutations associated with familial dilated cardiomyopathy

Protein	Gene	Locus	Mode of Transmission	Associated Phenotype	References
Sarcomeric					
Actin	ACTC	15q14	AD	None	22
α-tropomyosin	TPM1	15q22	AD	None	26
β-myosin heavy chain	MYH7	14q12	AD	None	23,31—33
α-myosin heavy chain	MYH6	14q12	AD	None	34
Troponin T	TNNT2	1q32	AD	None	23,25,35
Troponin C	TNNC1	3p21—p14	AD	None	25
Troponin I	TNNI3	19q13	AD, AR	None	36,37
Myosin-binding protein C	MYBPC3	11p11	AD	None	38
Sarcomere and Z-disc related					
Titin	TTN	2q31	AD	None	39
Telethonin	TCAP	17q12	AD	None	40,41
Muscle LIM protein	CSRP3	11p15	AD	None	40
Metavinculin	VCL	10q22—q23	AD	None	42
Cypher/ZASP	LDB3	10q22—q23	AD	CD, LVNC	43
α-Actinin 2	ACTN2	1q42—q43	AD	None	44
PDZ and LIM domain protein 3	PDLIM3	4q35	AD	None	45
Myopalladin	MYPN	10q21	AD	None	46
Four-and-a-half LIM protein 2	FHL2	2q12—q14	AD	None	47
Nexilin	NEXN	1p31	AD	None	48
Cytoskeletal					
Desmin	DES	2q35	AD	CD, SM	21,49
Dystrophin	DMD	Xp21	XLR	SM	20,50
δ-sarcoglycan	SGCD	5q33	AD	SD	18
αβ-crystallin	CRYAB	11q22—q23	AD	None	51
Nuclear					
Lamin A/C	LMNA	1q21	AD	CD, SD, SM	27,28,52—58
Thymopoeitin	TMPO	12q22	AD	None	59
Emerin	STA/EMD	Xq28	XLR	Emery-Dreifuss muscular dystrophy	60
Ion channel and ion channel—related					
Cardiac sodium channel	SCN5A	3p21	AD	CD	61,62
Sulphonylurea receptor-2 (SUR2)	ABCC9	12p12.1	AD	None	63
Desmosomal					
Desmoplakin	DSP	6p24	AR	Carvajal syndrome	64
Other					
Phospholamban	PLN	6q22	AD	None	65—67
Tafazzin	TAZ/G4.5	Xq28	XLR	Neutropenia, Short stature	68
M2 muscarinic receptor	CHRM2	7q35	AD#	CD, SD	69
Eya4	EYA4	6q23	AD#	SHL	70

(continued on next page)

Table 1
(continued)

Protein	Gene	Locus	Mode of Transmission	Associated Phenotype	References
LAMP2	*LAMP2*	Xq24	AD#	CD, SM	71
Laminin -α4	*LAMA4*	6q21	AD#	None	72
Integrin-linked kinase	*ILK*	11p15	AD#	None	72
Presenilin 1	*PSEN1*	14q24	AD#	None	73
Presenilin 2	*PSEN2*	1q31-q42	AD#	None	73
Cardiac ankyrin repeat protein (CARP)	*ANKRD1*	10q23	AD	None	74
RNA binding motif protein 20	*RBM20*	10q25	AD	None	75

Abbreviations: AD, autosomal dominant; AR, autosomal recessive; CD, conduction disease; LVNC, left ventricular non compaction; SD, sudden death; SHL, sensorineural hearing loss; SM, skeletal myopathy; XLR, X-linked recessive.

proportion of patients had a permanent pacemaker implanted, the risk of SCD remained high.

In a separate study, patients with *LMNA* mutations and conduction defects received an implantable cardioverter-defibrillator (ICD) instead of a pacemaker. Appropriate intervention for ventricular fibrillation or ventricular tachycardia (shock or antitachycardia pacing) was observed in 42% of these patients after a mean 34 months follow-up.[14] The mean LVEF in this cohort was 58%,

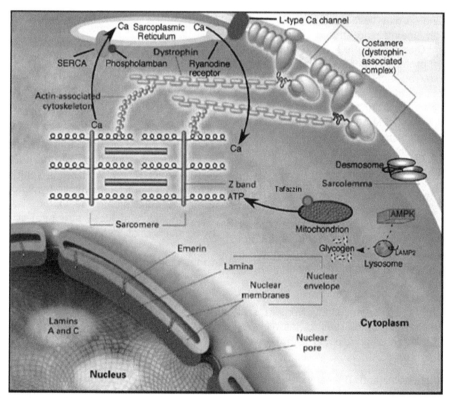

Fig. 1. The structure of the cardiac myocyte, showing the sarcomere, the cytoskeletal network, calcium channels, nuclear proteins, lysosomes, mitochondria, and AMP-activated protein kinase (AMPK). Mutations in the genes encoding most of the protein components of these structures lead to cardiomyopathies. *(From* Ahmad F, Seidman JG, Seidman CE. The genetic basis for cardiac remodeling. Annu Rev Genomics Hum Genet 2005;6:185–216; with permission.)

Table 2
Disease penetrance in autosomal dominant familial DCM

Age (y)	Clinical Disease Expression (%)
<20	10
20–29	35
30–39	60
>40	90

indicating a high risk of SCD before the development of significant DCM or cardiac failure.

Because reliable risk stratification in LMNA disease remains an unsolved challenge, consideration should be given to prophylactic ICD implantation in all patients who have a probable disease-causing mutation, particularly in the presence of a family history of premature SCD.

Desmosomal Disease

Mutations in desmosomal genes may cause a phenotype that resembles DCM. Desmosomes are cell adhesion junctions that are present in the epidermis and cardiac tissue and play an important role in maintaining tissue rigidity and strength.[89,90] Desmoplakin is the most abundant desmosomal protein. Loss of desmosomal integrity plays a key role in the pathogenesis of arrhythmogenic right ventricular cardiomyopathy (ARVC). Impaired cell-to-cell adhesion is purported to predispose to myocyte detachment and death, with fibro-fatty repair.

ARVC was originally described in young people presenting with arrhythmias of right ventricular origin, with fibro-fatty replacement of the right ventricular myocardium as the main pathologic feature. The right ventricle may be preferentially involved because of its thinner walls, which render it more susceptible to mechanical stress. Although left ventricular involvement is common in advanced disease, variants of ARVC with an early predilection for the left ventricle are also increasingly recognized.

The extent of left ventricle involvement and variations in the perceptible timing has allowed recognition of three distinct patterns of disease expression:

1. Classic (right dominant). The early stages of the disease are characterized by isolated right ventricular involvement, evolving from localized to diffuse. Left ventricular involvement may arise after the onset of global right ventricular dysfunction.

2. Left dominant, characterized by early prominent left ventricular involvement; the left ventricle is consistently more severely affected than the right.

3. Biventricular, characterized by parallel bilateral involvement with no apparent proclivity to either ventricle.

Left-dominant arrhythmogenic cardiomyopathy (LDAC) is characterized pathologically by fibroadipose replacement of the left ventricle, often occurring as a circumferential band in the outer one-third of the myocardium.[91–93] In classic right dominant disease, left ventricular involvement is frequently confined to the inferolateral and inferior walls, sparing the septum. LDAC, in contrast, affects the septum in more than 50% of cases. Cardiovascular magnetic resonance commonly shows late gadolinium enhancement in a subepicardial or midmyocardial distribution, consistent with that observed on pathology. Other structural changes include localized dilation, hypokinesia, or aneurysm formation.[94] In a study of 200 subjects with ARVC, 40% of the cohort had left ventricular abnormalities in the context of preserved right ventricular systolic function.[95]

Although LDAC is now accepted as a variant of ARVC, it can be clinically mistaken for DCM or myocarditis owing to its early and predominant left ventricular involvement. In one study, 50% of patients with confirmed LDAC had previously been misdiagnosed with viral myocarditis, DCM, hypertrophic cardiomyopathy, or idiopathic ventricular tachycardia.[96]

Another factor contributing to clinical underrecognition of LDAC may be the occurrence of histologic changes in the left ventricle in the absence of significant systolic dysfunction or left ventricular dilatation. This in turn leads to the underdetection of these structural abnormalities by conventional two-dimensional echocardiography. Other structural changes include right ventricular dysfunction and dilation, but the right ventricle is consistently less severely affected than the left.

The most common finding on a 12-lead ECG in subjects with LDAC is *T* wave inversion in the lateral or inferolateral leads, which may extend to the right precordial leads in a small number of patients, a pattern consistent with left ventricular predominance.[96] Ventricular arrhythmia can manifest as either ventricular tachycardia or frequent premature ventricular contractions on 24-hour ambulatory ECG monitoring or exercise testing. The typical right bundle branch block (BBB) morphology is consistent with left ventricular origin.[92,94,95] Arrhythmia of right ventricular origin (left BBB morphology) may also coexist, suggesting right ventricular involvement.

With recognition of disease subtypes with early left ventricular involvement, ARVC can no longer be defined by its right ventricular predilection, and adoption of the broader term *arrhythmogenic cardiomyopathy* has been proposed. Nonclassic subtypes of arrhythmogenic cardiomyopathy are differentiated from DCM on clinical grounds. One of the cardinal features of arrhythmogenic cardiomyopathy is a predisposition to ventricular arrhythmia that exceeds the degree of morphologic abnormality and ventricular dysfunction. In LDAC, for example, Sen-Chowdhry and colleagues[96] showed that the mean LVEF in patients with clinically significant ventricular arrhythmias was 54%. In contrast, both arrhythmic burden and risk in DCM caused by sarcomeric or cytoskeletal gene mutations are typically related to the severity of ventricular dysfunction.

DCM and arrhythmogenic cardiomyopathy also differ in the mode of clinical presentation. Heart failure is generally the first clinical manifestation of DCM, whereas in arrhythmogenic cardiomyopathy, the most common symptoms are palpitation and syncope. Symptoms are also a poor guide to disease severity in arrhythmogenic cardiomyopathy. No major differences are seen in most structural indices of the left and right ventricles between symptomatic and asymptomatic individuals.[95] In arrhythmogenic cardiomyopathy, most life-threatening events occur in apparently fit individuals with few or no symptoms,[13] and heart failure is a rare complication in survivors.

As with other subtypes of arrhythmogenic cardiomyopathy, LDAC is inherited in an autosomal dominant mode in most cases. The success rate from screening five desmosomal genes (*JUP*, *DSP*, *PKP2*, *DSG2*, and *DSC2*) in the LDAC cohort was approximately 30%.[96]

Autosomal recessive mode of inheritance is also described in Carvajal syndrome, a rare cardiocutaneous syndrome characterized by woolly hair, palmoplantar keratoderma, and left-dominant or biventricular subtype of arrhythmogenic cardiomyopathy. Cardiovascular manifestations include focal ventricular aneurysms,[64,97] ventricular tachyarrhythmias, and sudden death.[98]

GENETIC TESTING RECOMMENDATIONS

Current management practice in DCM is based on diagnostic and treatment algorithms that rarely consider potential differences in natural history and response to treatment in relation to the underlying genetic basis of the disease. In addition,

variation of age of onset, disease severity, and prognosis among members of families carrying the same causative mutation suggests that modifier genes also play a role in disease expression and, potentially, response to pharmacologic therapy. Current guidelines on the implantation of ICDs in patients with DCM are based mostly on large multicenter trials and registries of patients with impaired left ventricular function of any cause.

Screening for *LMNA* mutations should be considered in the presence of atrial fibrillation, conduction defects or skeletal myopathy, arrhythmic presentation, or a family history of sudden cardiac death in the absence of left ventricular systolic impairment and dilatation. Knowledge that a DCM patient is a carrier of an *LMNA* gene mutation is of major importance in deciding on device therapy. An upgrade to ICD is recommended in the presence of a conduction defect that requires the implantation of a permanent pacemaker (PPM), because the PPM may not prevent SCD. Implantation of an ICD is also recommended in patients with an *LMNA* mutation and a history of sustained ventricular tachycardia or aborted SCD, or a family history of SCD.

LDAC should be suspected in patients of any age with unexplained arrhythmia of left ventricular origin, (infero)lateral *T* wave inversion, apparent DCM (with arrhythmic presentation), or myocarditis (chest pain and enzyme rise with unobstructed coronary arteries). The significant risk of SCD in patients with LDAC justifies mutation screening for desmosomal genes in apparent DCM and warrants a low threshold for ICD placement if the diagnosis is confirmed.

DCM caused by gene mutations in proteins of the contractile apparatus and cytoskeleton are usually associated with symptoms of heart failure and left ventricular dysfunction, and primary ventricular arrhythmia is a rare presentation in these mutations. While mutations in the gene encoding the sodium channel (*SCN5A*) are associated with conduction defects and atrial fibrillation, ventricular arrhythmias are again uncommon in the absence of significant left ventricular dysfunction. Therefore, screening for these mutations has implications for family members but does not have significant implications on prognosis and treatment. Although comprehensive gene testing for mutations may become a part of the "state of the art" management, it cannot currently be recommended because of cost and other logistics of mutation analysis, which should improve within the next few years. However, unexpected sustained ventricular tachycardia or sudden death in the absence of significant left ventricular dysfunction should raise suspicion of either *LMNA* or a desmosomal mutation as the cause of the cardiomyopathy and should prompt familial evaluation.

REFERENCES

1. Codd MB, Sugrue DD, Gersh BJ, et al. Epidemiology of idiopathic dilated and hypertrophic cardiomyopathy. A population-based study in Olmsted County, Minnesota, 1975–1984. Circulation 1989; 80:564–72.
2. Manolio TA, Baughman KL, Rodeheffer R, et al. Prevalence and etiology of idiopathic dilated cardiomyopathy (summary of a national heart, lung, and blood institute workshop). Am J Cardiol 1992;69: 1458–66.
3. Hertz MI, Aurora P, Christie JD, et al. Scientific registry of the international society for heart and lung transplantation: introduction to the 2009 annual reports. J Heart Lung Transplant 2009;28:989–92.
4. Henry WL, Gardin JM, Ware JH. Echocardiographic measurements in normal subjects from infancy to old age. Circulation 1980;62:1054–61.
5. Baig MK, Goldman JH, Caforio AL, et al. Familial dilated cardiomyopathy: cardiac abnormalities are common in asymptomatic relatives and may represent early disease. J Am Coll Cardiol 1998;31: 195–201.
6. Caforio AL, Keeling PJ, Zachara E, et al. Evidence from family studies for autoimmunity in dilated cardiomyopathy. Lancet 1994;344:773–7.
7. Caforio AL, Mahon NG, Baig MK, et al. Prospective familial assessment in dilated cardiomyopathy: cardiac autoantibodies predict disease development in asymptomatic relatives. Circulation 2007; 115:76–83.
8. Mestroni L, Maisch B, McKenna WJ, et al. Guidelines for the study of familial dilated cardiomyopathies. Collaborative research group of the European human and capital mobility project on familial dilated cardiomyopathy. Eur Heart J 1999; 20:93–102.
9. Mahon NG, Murphy RT, MacRae CA, et al. Echocardiographic evaluation in asymptomatic relatives of patients with dilated cardiomyopathy reveals preclinical disease. Ann Intern Med 2005;143: 108–15.
10. Mahon NG, Madden BP, Caforio AL, et al. Immunohistologic evidence of myocardial disease in apparently healthy relatives of patients with dilated cardiomyopathy. J Am Coll Cardiol 2002;39:455–62.
11. Mahon NG, Sharma S, Elliott PM, et al. Abnormal cardiopulmonary exercise variables in asymptomatic relatives of patients with dilated cardiomyopathy who have left ventricular enlargement. Heart 2000;83: 511–7.
12. Gavazzi A, Repetto A, Scelsi L, et al. Evidence-based diagnosis of familial non-X-linked dilated cardiomyopathy. Prevalence, inheritance and characteristics. Eur Heart J 2001;22:73–81.
13. Mestroni L, Rocco C, Gregori D, et al. Familial dilated cardiomyopathy: evidence for genetic and phenotypic heterogeneity. Heart muscle disease study group. J Am Coll Cardiol 1999;34:181–90.
14. Meune C, Van Berlo JH, Anselme F, et al. Primary prevention of sudden death in patients with lamin A/C gene mutations. N Engl J Med 2006;354: 209–10.
15. Pasotti M, Klersy C, Pilotto A, et al. Long-term outcome and risk stratification in dilated cardiolaminopathies. J Am Coll Cardiol 2008;52:1250–60.
16. Van Berlo JH, de Voogt WG, van der Kooi AJ, et al. Meta-analysis of clinical characteristics of 299 carriers of LMNA gene mutations: do lamin A/C mutations portend a high risk of sudden death? J Mol Med 2005;83:79–83.
17. Ahmad F, Seidman JG, Seidman CE. The genetic basis for cardiac remodeling. Annu Rev Genomics Hum Genet 2005;6:185–216.
18. Tsubata S, Bowles KR, Vatta M, et al. Mutations in the human delta-sarcoglycan gene in familial and sporadic dilated cardiomyopathy. J Clin Invest 2000;106:655–62.
19. Barresi R, Di Blasi C, Negri T, et al. Disruption of heart sarcoglycan complex and severe cardiomyopathy caused by beta sarcoglycan mutations. J Med Genet 2000;37:102–7.
20. Arbustini E, Diegoli M, Morbini P, et al. Prevalence and characteristics of dystrophin defects in adult male patients with dilated cardiomyopathy. J Am Coll Cardiol 2000;35:1760–8.
21. Taylor MR, Slavov D, Ku L, et al. Prevalence of desmin mutations in dilated cardiomyopathy. Circulation 2007;115:1244–51.
22. Olson TM, Michels VV, Thibodeau SN, et al. Actin mutations in dilated cardiomyopathy, a heritable form of heart failure. Science 1998;280:750–2.
23. Kamisago M, Sharma SD, DePalma SR, et al. Mutations in sarcomere protein genes as a cause of dilated cardiomyopathy. N Engl J Med 2000;343: 1688–96.
24. Kaski JP, Burch M, Elliott PM. Mutations in the cardiac Troponin C gene are a cause of idiopathic dilated cardiomyopathy in childhood. Cardiol Young 2007;17:675–7.
25. Mogensen J, Murphy RT, Shaw T, et al. Severe disease expression of cardiac troponin C and T mutations in patients with idiopathic dilated cardiomyopathy. J Am Coll Cardiol 2004;44:2033–40.
26. Olson TM, Kishimoto NY, Whitby FG, et al. Mutations that alter the surface charge of alpha-tropomyosin are associated with dilated cardiomyopathy. J Mol Cell Cardiol 2001;33:723–32.

27. Fatkin D, MacRae C, Sasaki T, et al. Missense mutations in the rod domain of the lamin A/C gene as causes of dilated cardiomyopathy and conduction-system disease. N Engl J Med 1999; 341:1715–24.

28. Arbustini E, Pilotto A, Repetto A, et al. Autosomal dominant dilated cardiomyopathy with atrioventricular block: a lamin A/C defect-related disease. J Am Coll Cardiol 2002;39:981–90.

29. Bonne G, Di Barletta MR, Varnous S, et al. Mutations in the gene encoding lamin A/C cause autosomal dominant Emery-Dreifuss muscular dystrophy. Nat Genet 1999;21:285–8.

30. Arbustini E, Diegoli M, Fasani R, et al. Mitochondrial DNA mutations and mitochondrial abnormalities in dilated cardiomyopathy. Am J Pathol 1998;153:1501–10.

31. Daehmlow S, Erdmann J, Knueppel T, et al. Novel mutations in sarcomeric protein genes in dilated cardiomyopathy. Biochem Biophys Res Commun 2002;298:116–20.

32. Villard E, Duboscq-Bidot L, Charron P, et al. Mutation screening in dilated cardiomyopathy: prominent role of the beta myosin heavy chain gene. Eur Heart J 2005;26:794–803.

33. Karkkainen S, Helio T, Jaaskelainen P, et al. Two novel mutations in the beta-myosin heavy chain gene associated with dilated cardiomyopathy. Eur J Heart Fail 2004;6:861–8.

34. Carniel E, Taylor MR, Sinagra G, et al. Alpha-myosin heavy chain: a sarcomeric gene associated with dilated and hypertrophic phenotypes of cardiomyopathy. Circulation 2005;112:54–9.

35. Hanson EL, Jakobs PM, Keegan H, et al. Cardiac troponin T lysine 210 deletion in a family with dilated cardiomyopathy. J Card Fail 2002;8:28–32.

36. Murphy RT, Mogensen J, Shaw A, et al. Novel mutation in cardiac troponin I in recessive idiopathic dilated cardiomyopathy. Lancet 2004;363:371–2.

37. Carballo S, Robinson P, Otway R, et al. Identification and functional characterization of cardiac troponin I as a novel disease gene in autosomal dominant dilated cardiomyopathy. Circ Res 2009; 105:375–82.

38. Hershberger RE, Norton N, Morales A, et al. Coding sequence rare variants identified in MYBPC3, MYH6, TPM1, TNNC1, and TNNI3 from 312 patients with familial or idiopathic dilated cardiomyopathy. Circ Cardiovasc Genet 2010;3:155–61.

39. Gerull B, Gramlich M, Atherton J, et al. Mutations of TTN, encoding the giant muscle filament titin, cause familial dilated cardiomyopathy. Nat Genet 2002;30: 201–4.

40. Knoll R, Hoshijima M, Hoffman HM, et al. The cardiac mechanical stretch sensor machinery involves a Z disc complex that is defective in a subset of human dilated cardiomyopathy. Cell 2002;111:943–55.

41. Hayashi T, Arimura T, Itoh-Satoh M, et al. Tcap gene mutations in hypertrophic cardiomyopathy and dilated cardiomyopathy. J Am Coll Cardiol 2004; 44:2192–201.

42. Olson TM, Illenberger S, Kishimoto NY, et al. Meta-vinculin mutations alter actin interaction in dilated cardiomyopathy. Circulation 2002;105:431–7.

43. Vatta M, Mohapatra B, Jimenez S, et al. Mutations in Cypher/ZASP in patients with dilated cardiomyopathy and left ventricular non-compaction. J Am Coll Cardiol 2003;42:2014–27.

44. Mohapatra B, Jimenez S, Lin JH, et al. Mutations in the muscle LIM protein and alpha-actinin-2 genes in dilated cardiomyopathy and endocardial fibroelastosis. Mol Genet Metab 2003;80:207–15.

45. Arola AM, Sanchez X, Murphy RT, et al. Mutations in PDLIM3 and MYOZ1 encoding myocyte Z line proteins are infrequently found in idiopathic dilated cardiomyopathy. Mol Genet Metab 2007;90: 435–40.

46. Duboscq-Bidot L, Xu P, Charron P, et al. Mutations in the Z-band protein myopalladin gene and idiopathic dilated cardiomyopathy. Cardiovasc Res 2008;77: 118–25.

47. Arimura T, Hayashi T, Matsumoto Y, et al. Structural analysis of four and half LIM protein-2 in dilated cardiomyopathy. Biochem Biophys Res Commun 2007;357:162–7.

48. Hassel D, Dahme T, Erdmann J, et al. Nexilin mutations destabilize cardiac Z-disks and lead to dilated cardiomyopathy. Nat Med 2009;15:1281–8.

49. Li D, Tapscoft T, Gonzalez O, et al. Desmin mutation responsible for idiopathic dilated cardiomyopathy. Circulation 1999;100:461–4.

50. Towbin JA, Hejtmancik JF, Brink P, et al. X-linked dilated cardiomyopathy. Molecular genetic evidence of linkage to the Duchenne muscular dystrophy (dystrophin) gene at the Xp21 locus. Circulation 1993;87:1854–65.

51. Inagaki N, Hayashi T, Arimura T, et al. Alpha B-crystallin mutation in dilated cardiomyopathy. Biochem Biophys Res Commun 2006;342:379–86.

52. Brodsky GL, Muntoni F, Miocic S, et al. Lamin A/C gene mutation associated with dilated cardiomyopathy with variable skeletal muscle involvement. Circulation 2000;101:473–6.

53. Jakobs PM, Hanson EL, Crispell KA, et al. Novel lamin A/C mutations in two families with dilated cardiomyopathy and conduction system disease. J Card Fail 2001;7:249–56.

54. Vytopil M, Benedetti S, Ricci E, et al. Mutation analysis of the lamin A/C gene (LMNA) among patients with different cardiomuscular phenotypes. J Med Genet 2003;40:e132.

55. Taylor MR, Fain PR, Sinagra G, et al. Natural history of dilated cardiomyopathy due to lamin A/C gene mutations. J Am Coll Cardiol 2003;41:771–80.

56. Sylvius N, Bilinska ZT, Veinot JP, et al. In vivo and in vitro examination of the functional significances of novel lamin gene mutations in heart failure patients. J Med Genet 2005;42:639–47.

57. Sebillon P, Bouchier C, Bidot LD, et al. Expanding the phenotype of LMNA mutations in dilated cardiomyopathy and functional consequences of these mutations. J Med Genet 2003;40:560–7.

58. Burkett EL, Hershberger RE. Clinical and genetic issues in familial dilated cardiomyopathy. J Am Coll Cardiol 2005;45:969–81.

59. Taylor MR, Slavov D, Gajewski A, et al. Thymopoietin (lamina-associated polypeptide 2) gene mutation associated with dilated cardiomyopathy. Hum Mutat 2005;26:566–74.

60. Bione S, Small K, Aksmanovic VM, et al. Identification of new mutations in the Emery-Dreifuss muscular dystrophy gene and evidence for genetic heterogeneity of the disease. Hum Mol Genet 1995;4:1859–63.

61. McNair WP, Ku L, Taylor MR, et al. SCN5A mutation associated with dilated cardiomyopathy, conduction disorder, and arrhythmia. Circulation 2004;110:2163–7.

62. Olson TM, Michels VV, Ballew JD, et al. Sodium channel mutations and susceptibility to heart failure and atrial fibrillation. JAMA 2005;293:447–54.

63. Bienengraeber M, Olson TM, Selivanov VA, et al. ABCC9 mutations identified in human dilated cardiomyopathy disrupt catalytic KATP channel gating. Nat Genet 2004;36:382–7.

64. Norgett EE, Hatsell SJ, Carvajal-Huerta L, et al. Recessive mutation in desmoplakin disrupts desmoplakin-intermediate filament interactions and causes dilated cardiomyopathy, woolly hair and keratoderma. Hum Mol Genet 2000;9:2761–6.

65. Schmitt JP, Kamisago M, Asahi M, et al. Dilated cardiomyopathy and heart failure caused by a mutation in phospholamban. Science 2003;299:1410–3.

66. Haghighi K, Kolokathis F, Pater L, et al. Human phospholamban null results in lethal dilated cardiomyopathy revealing a critical difference between mouse and human. J Clin Invest 2003;111:869–76.

67. Haghighi K, Kolokathis F, Gramolini AO, et al. A mutation in the human phospholamban gene, deleting arginine 14, results in lethal, hereditary cardiomyopathy. Proc Natl Acad Sci U S A 2006;103:1388–93.

68. D'Adamo P, Fassone L, Gedeon A, et al. The X-linked gene G4.5 is responsible for different infantile dilated cardiomyopathies. Am J Hum Genet 1997;61:862–7.

69. Zhang L, Hu A, Yuan H, et al. A missense mutation in the CHRM2 gene is associated with familial dilated cardiomyopathy. Circ Res 2008;102:1426–32.

70. Schonberger J, Wang L, Shin JT, et al. Mutation in the transcriptional coactivator EYA4 causes dilated cardiomyopathy and sensorineural hearing loss. Nat Genet 2005;37:418–22.

71. Taylor MR, Ku L, Slavov D, et al. Danon disease presenting with dilated cardiomyopathy and a complex phenotype. J Hum Genet 2007;52:830–5.

72. Knoll R, Postel R, Wang J, et al. Laminin-alpha4 and integrin-linked kinase mutations cause human cardiomyopathy via simultaneous defects in cardiomyocytes and endothelial cells. Circulation 2007;116:515–25.

73. Li D, Parks SB, Kushner JD, et al. Mutations of presenilin genes in dilated cardiomyopathy and heart failure. Am J Hum Genet 2006;79:1030–9.

74. Moulik M, Vatta M, Witt SH, et al. ANKRD1, the gene encoding cardiac ankyrin repeat protein, is a novel dilated cardiomyopathy gene. J Am Coll Cardiol 2009;54:325–33.

75. Brauch KM, Karst ML, Herron KJ, et al. Mutations in ribonucleic acid binding protein gene cause familial dilated cardiomyopathy. J Am Coll Cardiol 2009;54:930–41.

76. Kass S, MacRae C, Graber HL, et al. A gene defect that causes conduction system disease and dilated cardiomyopathy maps to chromosome 1p1-1q1. Nat Genet 1994;7:546–51.

77. Messina DN, Speer MC, Pericak-Vance MA, et al. Linkage of familial dilated cardiomyopathy with conduction defect and muscular dystrophy to chromosome 6q23. Am J Hum Genet 1997;61:909–17.

78. Elliott P, Andersson B, Arbustini E, et al. Classification of the cardiomyopathies: a position statement from the European society of cardiology working group on myocardial and pericardial diseases. Eur Heart J 2008;29:270–6.

79. Felice KJ, Schwartz RC, Brown CA, et al. Autosomal dominant Emery-Dreifuss dystrophy due to mutations in rod domain of the lamin A/C gene. Neurology 2000;55:275–80.

80. Speckman RA, Garg A, Du F, et al. Mutational and haplotype analyses of families with familial partial lipodystrophy (Dunnigan variety) reveal recurrent missense mutations in the globular C-terminal domain of lamin A/C. Am J Hum Genet 2000;66:1192–8.

81. Shackleton S, Lloyd DJ, Jackson SN, et al. LMNA, encoding lamin A/C, is mutated in partial lipodystrophy. Nat Genet 2000;24:153–6.

82. Muchir A, Bonne G, van der Kooi AJ, et al. Identification of mutations in the gene encoding lamins A/C in autosomal dominant limb girdle muscular dystrophy with atrioventricular conduction disturbances (LGMD1B). Hum Mol Genet 2000;9:1453–9.

83. De Backer J, Van Beeumen K, Loeys B, et al. Expanding the phenotype of sudden cardiac death—an unusual presentation of a family with a lamin A/C mutation. Int J Cardiol 2010;138:97–9.

84. Rober RA, Weber K, Osborn M. Differential timing of nuclear lamin A/C expression in the various organs of the mouse embryo and the young animal: a developmental study. Development 1989;105:365–78.

85. Fisher DZ, Chaudhary N, Blobel G. cDNA sequencing of nuclear lamins A and C reveals primary and secondary structural homology to intermediate filament proteins. Proc Natl Acad Sci U S A 1986;83:6450–4.

86. Gerace L, Blobel G. The nuclear envelope lamina is reversibly depolymerized during mitosis. Cell 1980; 19:277–87.

87. Nikolova V, Leimena C, McMahon AC, et al. Defects in nuclear structure and function promote dilated cardiomyopathy in lamin A/C-deficient mice. J Clin Invest 2004;113:357–69.

88. Becane HM, Bonne G, Varnous S, et al. High incidence of sudden death with conduction system and myocardial disease due to lamins A and C gene mutation. Pacing Clin Electrophysiol 2000;23:1661–6.

89. Smith EA, Fuchs E. Defining the interactions between intermediate filaments and desmosomes. J Cell Biol 1998;141:1229–41.

90. Gallicano GI, Kouklis P, Bauer C, et al. Desmoplakin is required early in development for assembly of desmosomes and cytoskeletal linkage. J Cell Biol 1998;143:2009–22.

91. Gallo P, D'Amati G, Pelliccia F. Pathologic evidence of extensive left ventricular involvement in arrhythmogenic right ventricular cardiomyopathy. Hum Pathol 1992;23:948–52.

92. De Pasquale CG, Heddle WF. Left sided arrhythmogenic ventricular dysplasia in siblings. Heart 2001; 86:128–30.

93. Michalodimitrakis M, Papadomanolakis A, Stiakakis J, et al. Left side right ventricular cardiomyopathy. Med Sci Law 2002;42:313–7.

94. Norman M, Simpson M, Mogensen J, et al. Novel mutation in desmoplakin causes arrhythmogenic left ventricular cardiomyopathy. Circulation 2005; 112:636–42.

95. Sen-Chowdhry S, Syrris P, Ward D, et al. Clinical and genetic characterization of families with arrhythmogenic right ventricular dysplasia/cardiomyopathy provides novel insights into patterns of disease expression. Circulation 2007;115:1710–20.

96. Sen-Chowdhry S, Syrris P, Prasad SK, et al. Left-dominant arrhythmogenic cardiomyopathy: an under-recognized clinical entity. J Am Coll Cardiol 2008;52:2175–87.

97. Kaplan SR, Gard JJ, Carvajal-Huerta L, et al. Structural and molecular pathology of the heart in Carvajal syndrome. Cardiovasc Pathol 2004;13:26–32.

98. Alcalai R, Metzger S, Rosenheck S, et al. A recessive mutation in desmoplakin causes arrhythmogenic right ventricular dysplasia, skin disorder, and woolly hair. J Am Coll Cardiol 2003; 42:319–27.

Genetic Testing for Cardiac Arrhythmias: Ready for Prime Time?

Steven J. Fowler, MD[a,b], Raffaella Bloise, MD[c,d],*

KEYWORDS

- Genetics • Cardiac • Arrhythmias • Channelopathies
- Multidisciplinary approach

The identification of genetic bases of inherited arrhythmogenic diseases (IAD) has facilitated a progressive understanding of their pathophysiology[1,2] and has given to the clinician new facilities for genetic-based risk stratification and therapy.[3] Genetic analysis can be performed to identify the molecular substrate in those patients affected or suspected to be affected by an inherited arrhythmogenic disease; however, the clinical usefulness of this information is often not straightforward and it requires specific expertise and a multidisciplinary teamwork by the cardiologist, the clinical geneticist, and the molecular biologist. Of importance, growing epidemiologic evidence supports the idea that knowing the type of DNA abnormality is not merely a "molecular afterthought" to the clinical diagnosis, but may play a key part in the care of these unique patients: but are we ready for them to play a prime-time role?

Despite the heterogeneity of substrates and clinical expressivity, genetic testing has a direct impact on clinical practice: it allows a specific diagnosis, including silent carriers (ie, asymptomatic diagnosis) and, in select diseases, the identification of a mutation has major impact for risk stratification and treatment of patients.[3] The following overview addresses the role of genetic testing for each of the most epidemiologically relevant inherited arrhythmogenic diseases, specifically Long QT Syndrome (LQTS), Brugada Syndrome (BrS), Catecholaminergic Polymorphic Ventricular Tachycardia (CPVT), Hypertrophic Cardiomyopathy (HCM), and Arrhythmogenic Right Ventricular Cardiomyopathy (ARVC).

LONG QT SYNDROME

LQTS is characterized by abnormally prolonged ventricular repolarization and increased risk of malignant ventricular tachyarrhythmias, in patients with a morphologically intact heart.[4] The estimated prevalence is between 1:2500 and 1:5000. However, given that up to two-thirds of patients are probably missed,[5] that 10% to 35% of LQTS patients present with a normal QTc interval, and that there may a delay to diagnosis via misclassification as epilepsy,[6] it is likely that the actual prevalence is higher. The mean age at onset of symptoms (syncope or sudden death) is 12 years, and an earlier onset is usually associated with a more severe outcome.[7]

LQTS is associated with sudden cardiac death, therefore it is listed among the life-threatening diseases; what is rather unusual is that when the proper diagnosis is established, the most severe complications can be prevented with the use of anti-adrenergic treatments (β-blocker therapy) and, in severe cases, with Implantable Cardioverter-Defibrillator (ICD) insertion. The ability of clinicians to recognize and treat the disease is extremely effective in preventing casualties in patients. It is

[a] Cardiovascular Genetics Program, Leon H. Charney Division of Cardiology, NYU Langone Medical Center, New York, USA
[b] Clinical Cardiac Electrophysiology, Leon H. Charney Division of Cardiology, NYU Langone Medical Center, New York, USA
[c] Molecular Cardiology, IRCCS Fondazione Salvatore Maugeri, Pavia, Italy
[d] Department of Cardiology, University of Pavia, Pavia, Italy
* Corresponding author. Molecular Cardiology, IRCCS Fondazione Salvatore Maugeri, Pavia, Italy.
E-mail address: raffaella.bloise@fsm.it

Card Electrophysiol Clin 2 (2010) 611–621
doi:10.1016/j.ccep.2010.10.001
1877-9182/10/$ — see front matter © 2010 Published by Elsevier Inc.

therefore of major relevance that clinical cardiologists, pediatricians, neurologists, and sport physicians are able to recognize LQTS and to refer patients to specialized centers.

Genetic Analysis in LQTS

LQTS is transmitted mainly as an autosomal dominant disease, Romano-Ward syndrome (R-W), which accounts for the majority of cases. The autosomal recessive form denominated Jervell and Lange-Nielsen syndrome (J-LN) is characterized by the coexistence of QT prolongation and congenital deafness.

The list of LQTS-causing genes is continuously expanding, and has reached a current count of 12 candidates (**Table 1**). LQTS genes affect ionic currents, either directly (ion channel mutations) or indirectly (chaperones and/or other modulators), and it is now clear that nonion channel encoding genes may also cause the disease.[8] Two forms, LQT7 and LQT8, are characterized by the presence of an extracardiac phenotype resulting in 2 distinct syndromes. LQT7 (Andersen syndrome), caused by mutations on *KCNJ2* gene, is a rare variant (<1%): it includes periodic paralysis of the legs and dysmorphic features. The electrocardiogram of the affected patients is characterized by the presence of marked U waves and ventricular arrhythmias including bidirectional ventricular tachycardia.[9] LQT8 (Timothy syndrome), caused by mutations on *CACNA1C* gene, presents an extremely severe phenotype, including QT prolongation, syndactyly, congenital heart defects,

autism, reduced immune response, and developmental disorders.[10]

A genetic defect is identified in from 60% to 72% (variable in different laboratories) of LQTS patients,[11] suggesting that still a significant percentage of the patients have mutations on unknown genes. Genetic heterogeneity in LQTS is remarkable, but 3 genes dominate the picture: *KCNQ1* (LQT1), *KCNH2* (LQT2), and *SCN5A* (LQT3) cover more than 90% of LQTS patients with identified mutations.[12] This observation is relevant in terms of genetic testing because it implies that comprehensive screening of at least major genes should always be performed given the correct clinical context: electrocardiogram (ECG) findings, personal and family history, and symptomatology.[13] Moreover, the probability of positive genotyping is highest (up to 72%) when performed in those with the highest phenotypic probability of having the syndrome,[14–16] further enforcing the role of phenotype correlation guiding rational genotyping decisions.

The screening on *ANK2*, *KCNJ2*, and *CACNA1C* is performed only in the presence of the specific clinical features. The genotype has a direct clinical impact in LQTS: gene-specific differences have been described in terms of morphology of the ST-T wave complex, triggers for cardiac events,[17] and risk of cardiac events.[7,18,19] Genotype-phenotype studies have provided important information regarding the effect of location, coding type, and biophysical function of the channel mutations on the phenotypic manifestations and clinical course of LQTS patients.[20] Based on these

Table 1
Distinguishing features of different LQTS forms

Syndrome	Inheritance	Gene(s)	Phenotype
Romano-Ward	Dominant	KCNQ1, KCNH2, SCN5A, CaV3, ANK2, AKAP9, KCNE1, KCNE2, SCN4B	Isolated QT prolongation and abnormal repolarization morphology
Jervell and Lange-Nielsen	Recessive	KCNQ1, KCNE1	Markedly prolonged QT interval and deafness
Andersen-Tawil	Dominant	KCNJ2	Hypokalemic periodic paralysis, facial dysmorphism, prolonged QT with giant U wave
Timothy syndrome	Only sporadic cases, reported parental mosaicism	CACNA1C	Markedly prolonged QT interval, syndactyly, congenital heart defects, autism, hypoglycemia, recurrent infections

findings, there is consensus that LQT2 and LQT3 genotypes show a worse prognosis and relatively poor response to β-blocker therapy. With regard to treatment in genotyped patients, β-blocker therapy has been associated with a significant reduction in the rate of cardiac events in patients with LQT1 and LQT2 mutations, but no evident reduction in those with LQT3 mutations.[21] ICD implant for the primary prevention of sudden cardiac arrest may be considered in these LQTS variants when associated with QTc greater than 500 ms and an early onset of cardiac events (<7 years of age). It can be concluded that the locus of the causative mutation affects the clinical course in LQTS and modulates the effects of the QTc, along with gender, on clinical manifestations. Based on these data, the authors' group proposed an approach to risk stratification based on these variables (**Fig. 1**).

Moving further toward mutation-specific risk assessment, data regarding cardiac event rates with respect to the location of mutations has shown that *KCNH2 pore* mutations are independent predictors of a malignant outcome whereas *KCNQ1* C−terminal mutations are independent predictors of a benign prognosis.[20,22] The dominant-negative *KCNQ1*-A341 V mutation (>50% loss of I_{ks} current) is associated with a particularly high clinical severity independent of ethnicity.[23,24] Additional evidence suggests that biophysical characterization of mutants may also provide important clues; for example, the authors' group has demonstrated that the clinical response to mexiletine (a gene-specific therapy for LQT3) may be predicted on the basis of in vitro characterization of the underlying *SCN5A* mutation (discussed in greater detail later in this article). From this brief overview, it is clear to see how genotyping can make a significant clinical impact in the care plan for LQTS patients, and is indeed ready for prime time.

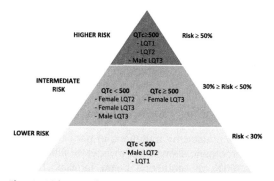

Fig. 1. Risk stratification for LQTS. (*From* Priori SG, Schwartz PJ, Napolitano C, et al. Risk stratification in the long-QT syndrome. N Engl J Med 2003;348: 1866–74; with permission.)

BRUGADA SYNDROME

BrS is an inherited arrhythmogenic disease characterized by a unique electrocardiographic pattern of ST segment elevation in leads V_1 to V_3, and incomplete or complete right bundle branch block in the absence of acute myocardial ischemia; it is characterized clinically by syncope and sudden death resulting from episodes of polymorphic ventricular tachycardia.[25] The disease is inherited with autosomal dominant pattern, but there is a male to female ratio of 8:1. The estimated worldwide prevalence is of 0.10%,[26] and it may exceed this figure in endemic areas of Southeast Asia.[27]

Genetic Analysis in BrS

The first identified gene for BrS (BrS1) is *SCN5A*,[28] encoding for the α-subunit of the cardiac sodium channel protein (NaV1.5). Unlike the LQT3 subtype of LQTS, which involves a gain of function *SCN5A* mutation, BrS1 mutations cause a loss of function.[29] Now, more than 90 *SCN5A* mutations are linked to BrS:BrS1 patients account for 18% to 30% of clinically diagnosed cases.[30] It is clear that approximately two-thirds of Brugada patients have not yet been genotyped, suggesting the presence of substantial genetic heterogeneity.[31] Approximately 65% of mutations identified in *SCN5A* gene are associated with a BrS phenotype. However, prior sudden death events, syncope, spontaneous development of a type 1 pattern, and inducibility during programmed electrical stimulation (PES) serve as the strongest predictors of ongoing risk.[32]

The BrS2 gene is *GPD1-L*, encoding for the glycerol-3-phosphate-dehydrogenase-1like protein[33]: mutations in *GPD1-L* decrease *SCN5A* surface membrane expression and reduces I_{Na}. Two other genes involved in BrS are *CACNA1C* (BrS3) and *CACNB2* (BrS4), the gene encoding the α1- and β2b-subunit of the L-type calcium channel, respectively, discovered in 3 probands with Brugada ST-segment elevation associated with a short QT interval[34] caused by loss of function of I_{Ca-L}. *SCN1B* that encodes for the function-modifying subunit (β1) of the cardiac sodium channel is the cause of BrS5 in a family with BrS and cardiac conduction disease.[35] BrS6 is a rare variant, identified so far in only one single family with a mutation of *KCNE3* gene encoding for the MiRP potassium channel subunit: mutations on this gene cause an increase in the I_{to} current, as well as an accelerated inactivation.[36] Finally, BrS7 gene, *SCN3B* (encoding for the β3 subunit of the cardiac sodium channel), has been recently identified in a single patient[37]: it influences the function of Nav1.5, controlling the intracellular trafficking of the sodium channel.

Because the relative prevalence of mutations on the other genes related to BrS is unknown (and likely very low), the routine screening of these genes, with the exception of SCN5A, has an uncertain diagnostic value. Of note, patient carriers of SCN5A mutations often present a concomitant conduction defect: as a consequence prolonged PR and/or prolonged HV interval are phenotypical features of Brs1.[38] By extension, the presence of late potentials should be regarded as a clinical marker of the disease, as they occur in some 50% of clinically affected patients.

A possible explanation of the race-specific differential prevalence of the BrS phenotype has been suggested by Bezzina and colleagues[39] after observing the presence of an Asian-specific haplotype (high frequency of 0.22): a 6 single-nucleotide polymorphism (SNP) block not present among Caucasians, causing lower transcription activity of the gene, clinically associated with a reduced intraventricular conduction velocity. Analysis has also demonstrated that prolonged PR duration correlates to both SCN5A mutation status and inducibility of ventricular tachycardia or ventricular fibrillation during PES.[40,41] Incidence of supraventricular tachycardia—predominantly atrial fibrillation—is approximately 20%, and these arrhythmias are more likely to be present in those requiring an ICD.[42]

Due to the complexity of the biophysical abnormalities caused by SCN5A mutations, overlapping phenotypes between BrS, LQT3, progressive cardiac conduction defects and sick sinus syndrome have been reported.[29,43–45] Furthermore, SCN5A mutations can be associated with myocardial abnormalities similar to those observed in ARVC[46,47] and in dilated cardiomyopathy (DCM).[48] These clinical overlaps make a precise genotype-phenotype correlation challenging for physicians, who need to keep an open mind when assessing for arrhythmogenic diseases related to SCN5A; taken in this context, genetic testing can play a prime-time role in Brugada syndrome.

CATECHOLAMINERGIC POLYMORPHIC VENTRICULAR TACHYCARDIA

CPVT is a disorder of intracellular calcium handling,[49] characterized by adrenergic-dependent arrhythmias. The estimated prevalence is 1:7000 to 1:10,000, and the mortality rate in untreated individuals approaches 50% by age 40.[50] CPVT patients display an unremarkable resting ECG with the exception of sinus bradycardia, absence of structural heart disease, and exercise or emotion-induced syncopal events with a distinctive pattern of bidirectional ventricular tachycardia during exercise or catecholamine infusion.[51]

Genetic Analysis in CPVT

Mutations in the cardiac ryanodine receptor gene (hRyR2) and calsequestrin gene (CASQ2) are respectively responsible for the autosomal dominant and recessive variants of CPVT.[52,53] Some 70% of genotyped patients carry a mutation on the hRyR2 gene,[50] while the prevalence of CASQ2 mutations is low (~7% in the authors' cohort).[54] Genetic analysis is logistically complicated by the fact that hRYR2 is one of the largest genes in the human genome, and genotyping turnaround time is long. As with other inherited forms of cardiac arrhythmia, CPVT involves a high degree of genetic heterogeneity. Therefore, mutation scanning of the open reading frame regions of hRyR2 and CASQ2 is the best approach for mutation detection respect to targeted exon analysis.

A coherent hRyR2/CASQ2 screening approach has to include 2 additional important observations: first, 20% of mutation carriers have no phenotype (incomplete penetrance) and second, sudden cardiac arrest can be the first clinical presentation of the disease in up to 62%.[54] Therefore, CPVT may be regarded as a cause of adrenergically mediated idiopathic ventricular fibrillation (IVF), justifying genetic testing in such instances.

Anecdotal reports show that KCNJ2 (LQT7) mutations may cause a CPVT phenotype.[55] This point is particularly important to consider for hRyR2 and CASQ2-negative patients, because KCNJ2 mutations are usually associated with a more benign prognosis, and sudden death is considered an exceptional event in these cases.[9] Thus, molecular diagnosis may provide important prognostic insight in these cases.

Early CPVT genetic evaluation is very important for all family members of CPVT probands, for presymptomatic diagnosis and appropriate reproductive counseling. Furthermore, as β-blockers are often an effective treatment, genetic diagnosis of CPVT is relevant in the prevention of life-threatening events, improving prognosis substantially,[50] and worthy of prime-time status.

HYPERTROPHIC CARDIOMYOPATHY

HCM is caused by mutations in genes encoding the sarcomeric elements of myocytes, with greater than 90% of mutations being familial. Though the most prevalent (0.2%, 1:500)[56] and thus the most reported and investigated of heritable cardiomyopathies, the classification of sudden cardiac death (SCD) risk predictors and prognosis for HCM remains difficult and has not been definitively established. Severe clinical conditions such as heart failure, supraventricular and ventricular arrhythmias, and SCD are possible.

The histopathological hallmarks of HCM are marked myocyte hypertrophy, fibrosis, and disarray, reflecting the underlying pathophysiology of impaired ventricular contractility. Comparative functional analysis of HCM myomectomy samples and end-stage heart failure samples has revealed a common molecular phenotype demonstrating deranged myosin phosphorylation, impaired motility, and reduced contraction amplitude and relaxation rates, irrespective of genotype.[57] Noninvasive predictors of SCD risk include SCD in first-degree relatives, malignant genotype, unexplained syncope, abnormal blood pressure response to exercise, ectopic ventricular activity, and massive septal hypertrophy ($\geq$30 mm),[58] with new data incorporating scar by delayed-enhancement cardiac magnetic resonance to correlate to arrhythmic events.[59]

Genetic Analysis in HCM

To date, more than 450 mutations in 21 sarcomere-related and myofilament-related genes have been identified in HCM.[60] Mutations in the genes encoding the beta-myosin heavy chain (*MYH7*), myosin-binding protein C (*MYBPC3*), and cardiac troponin-T (*TNNT2*) are responsible for more than 45% of familial HCM, and 88% of disease-causing genes reside on these 3 loci.[60] Analogous to what has been described for other inherited arrhythmogenic diseases, the consequence of mutations varies in different carriers (incomplete penetrance and variable expressivity). What determines the severity of clinical manifestations in response to a mutation is not known; the role of both causal mutations and modifier genes and/or factors in the ultimate pattern of clinical expression has been suggested.[61] This heterogeneity makes the direct use of genotyping less clinically applicable outside of a specific phenotype.

Considering the complex genotype-phenotype correlations, genetic screening is the only method that may enable the recognition of mutation carriers in the preclinical phase of the disease. Genotyping may also help to distinguish pathologic from normal variants, such as the athletic heart, hypertensive heart disease, or asymmetric septal hypertrophy. Appropriate clinical evaluation before testing is key to eliminating the rare nonsarcomeric variants, termed "phenocopies" (ie, Noonan syndrome, Friedrich ataxia, Anderson-Fabry disease, amyloidosis, and so forth), in which thickening of the left ventricular wall resembling

HCM can occur,[62] as a consequence of metabolic disorders or mitochondrial cytopathies. Phenocopies tend to express more conduction disease and progression to cavitary dilatation and heart failure, and extracardiac manifestations can be present.[63]

Some genotype-phenotype correlations have been reported for HCM causing mutations. *MYH7* mutations, like A403G and A453C, often create highly penetrant disease phenotypes with severe myocardial hypertrophy at a young age, heart failure, and unfavorable prognosis for SCD.[64] However, there are other mutations, located on the same gene, that portend a more favorable prognosis (ie, N232S, G256E, V403Q), with less hypertrophy and less reported symptomatology. These major allelic differences in disease expression have been attributed to the electric charge of the missense amino acid or to the specific β-subunit affected, but need to be substantiated.[65]

Because of the high yield of analysis for HCM, in which approximately 90% of patients with an identifiable mutation may be identified by screening only 4 of the 21 known genes, genotyping is recommended for the most affected individual in a given family in order to facilitate family screening and to guide exact disease management.[66] A reasonable expectation for positive genotyping is about 60% of affected patients, with *MYH7*, *MYBPC3*, and *TNNT2* accounting for 25% to 35%, 20% to 30%, and 3% to 5%, respectively[67]; with an understanding that genotyping is clearly not ready for prime time unless driven by a specific clinical scenario.

ARRHYTHMOGENIC RIGHT VENTRICULAR CARDIOMYOPATHY

ARVC is a disorder of the cardiac desmosome, a protein responsible for supporting structural stability through cell-cell adhesion, regulating transcription of genes involved in adipogenesis and apoptosis, and maintaining proper electrical conductivity through regulation of gap junctions and calcium homeostasis.[68] The estimated prevalence of the disease is 1:5000; it is thought to be a major contributor to SCD in young people and athletes worldwide, with a mortality rate of 2% to 4% annually.[69] ARVC is a predominantly autosomal dominant disease characterized by myocardial degeneration and fibrofatty infiltration of the right ventricular free wall, the subtricuspid region, and the outflow tract. A rare, autosomal recessive variant (Naxos disease) characterized by typical myocardial involvement, palmar keratosis, and woolly hair has also been described.[70] The histopathophysiology of ARVC involves the progressive replacement of myocardial tissue with fibro-fatty tissue, predominantly in the right ventricle, but often also involving the left ventricle (in up to 25%), resulting in malignant arrhythmia of ventricular origin.[71]

Genetic Analysis in ARVC

Mutation in genes encoding any of the 5 major components of the desmosome can result in ARVC, but PKP2 (encoding plakophilin-2), DSG2 (encoding desmoglein-2), and DSP (encoding desmoplakin) account for the majority: 27%, 26%, and 11% of mutations, respectively.[72] In pooled analysis, 39.2% of individuals with ARVC who have undergone full sequence analysis of all the desmosome genes have a single, heterozygous mutation identified.[73] At present, as is the case with HCM, there is no clear risk stratification that may be gleaned from genotyping ARVC; recent literature has shown that PKP2 genotype–positive patients have symptom and arrhythmia onset at an earlier age, but prospective defibrillator events were not significantly different from the PKP2 negative cohort.[74]

Enabling cascade screening in relatives becomes the principal issue, as it may avert a lifetime of clinical reassessment in extended ARVC families; therefore, genotyping in ARVC may be recommended for confirmation of select index cases. First-degree relatives should be screened clinically with 12-lead ECG, echocardiography, and cardiac magnetic resonance imaging; genotyping is not ready for a first-line, prime-time slot. The ARVC Task Force clinical criteria, in the final process of being updated, provide the best diagnostic tool for ARVC screening.[75]

GENETIC COUNSELING

Genetic counseling is a medical action aimed to help patients and their families deal with the problems related to the diagnosis of a genetic disease. With the increased use of genetic testing, genetic counseling has become a fundamental part of the process; it is important to give the patients autonomy in their choice. Genetic counseling should be performed by professionals with particular training, who are prepared to give support to the patient and his family whatever will be their decision.[76] In fact, genetic counseling primarily serves an informational and not a directive purpose: in particular, it helps patients understand the diagnosis, hereditary pattern, implications, and therapeutic possibilities to avoid recurrence of the disease. A genetic counselor gives information to improve the quality of life and health of affected subjects, with particular sensitivity to their genetic nature; and by extension, counseling patients to communicate to the extended family the importance of screening for high-risk inherited disease.[77]

In some cases the benefits gained from identifying a pathogenic mutation can be substantial; in others the same discovery could have important negative effects. In particular, detecting mutations that portend an increased risk of sudden death, in absence of a therapy, can present a family with complex and difficult issues to consider, ranging from medical (ie, clinical management), legal (ie, insurance), and social (ie, lifestyle, family planning, stigmatization), to psychological (ie, feelings of anxiety or guilt). Genotyping may not be appropriate for every case of IAD, and a decision whether to offer analysis should be made within the context of and with the cooperation of each unique family. In particular, presymptomatic testing, in particular in minors, should be carefully evaluated, under strict cooperation of the cardiologist and the genetic counselor with the parents. Such considerations would accordingly preclude the inappropriate "blanket" genotype testing for those with an undefined condition.

CURRENT LIMITATIONS OF GENETIC TESTING

In only a handful of years, genetic testing for inherited arrhythmogenic diseases has emerged from the research laboratory into commercial testing, making this service more accessible to the medical community. While in principle this is a positive advancement, it is also clear that it poses some issues: the interpretation of genetic findings is often not straightforward.

The identification of a previously reported mutation with clear cosegregation evidence, high penetrance and, even more, with known biophysical consequences (in vitro expression data), is very helpful for clinical management. On the other hand, the identification of novel mutants in sporadic cases or in families with low penetrance, in the absence of functional information, generates uncertainties in interpretation, and requires evaluation in tertiary centers with specific expertise and experience in diagnosis and treatment of inherited arrhythmogenic disorders and cardiovascular genetics.

Aforementioned factors that limit the current clinical applicability of genetic testing are: low prevalence of a specific genetic variant preventing the collection of adequate study cohorts for genotype-phenotype correlation studies; variability of phenotype in subjects with the same genetic defect; large deletions; and polymorphisms and

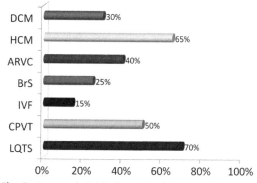

Fig. 2. Expected yield of genotyping.

gene modifiers. The advancement in understanding these cofactors remains crucial to allow a prime-time role for genotyping (**Fig. 2** and **Table 2**).

Cost Considerations

The science used in genotyping and mutational analysis bears considerable financial costs, although progressively diminishing as technique and technology advance. Reimbursement policies dealing with this issue are universally lacking, an impediment prohibiting further incorporation into clinical practice. Recently published data regarding cost effectiveness[78] outlines that genotyping can be performed at reasonable cost in individuals with a conclusive diagnosis—specifically, LQTS, CPVT, and BrS with atrioventricular block; a fact that would likely extend to both HCM and ARVC, though not presented.

It is clear that careful phenotyping through disease and patient specific correlations are the key to controlling costs; arriving at a genetic diagnosis is not synonymous with simply ordering

a test. Moreover, the integrated expertise of a cardiogenetics team is best suited for the labor-, time-, and resource-intensive longitudinal care that necessarily ensues following a positive diagnosis of an inherited arrhythmogenic disease.

BEYOND DNA SEQUENCING

Recent literature hints at the future of integrating genotyping into clinical practice: applying results of functional characterization to the clinical management.

Patient-Specific In Vitro Definition of Clinical Effectiveness

Based on evidence that LQT3 is caused by an increase of inward sodium current leading to prolongation of the action potential duration, the use of sodium channel blockers has been proposed as a gene-specific therapy and has been evaluated in the clinical setting.[79,80] Taking into account the ensuing clinical observation that not all carriers of *SCN5A* mutations responded to sodium channel blockers with a significant shortening of repolarization, the authors advanced and tested the hypothesis that biophysical properties of mutants could help identify LQT3 patients who would benefit most from treatment.

The authors selected 5 LQT3 probands with documented ventricular tachyarrhythmias before therapy who were treated with mexiletine. Over a mean follow-up of 4.6 years on mexiletine, 3 probands who responded to mexiletine with a QTc shortening remained free from cardiac events. Two patients who had negligible or no QTc shortening died of sudden cardiac arrest during mexiletine therapy. The authors then extensively characterized the biophysical properties of the mutant channels. The results suggested that

Table 2
Application possibilities of genotyping

	Silent Carriers/Diagnosis	Reproductive Risk Assessment	Prognosis	Therapy
LQTS	+	+	+	+
CPVT	+	+	±	±
SQTS	+	+	−	−
BrS	+	+	−	−
IVF	+	+	−	−
ARVC	+	+	−	−
Lamin A/C	+	+	+	−
DCM	+	+	−	−
HCM	+	+	−	−

a negative V1/2 shift of steady-state inactivation (SSI) and different mutation-specific EC_{50} for use-dependent block is invariably associated with good clinical response to mexiletine.[81]

In a related study, the authors further the concept that despite the "average" behavior of patients with mutations in a given gene being uncovered by phenotype-genotype correlation, the next challenge is to delineate "mutation-specific" characteristics. The authors identified a child with marked QT prolongation and recurrent polymorphic VT and VF who was carrier of a de novo *SCN5A* mutation, which causes the appearance of large sustained sodium current but also a reduction of peak current density; the latter being a typical feature of Brugada syndrome. Clinically, therapy with mexiletine was observed to be detrimental in this individual, dramatically increasing arrhythmias. Subsequent in vitro functional characterization study of the mutation revealed that mexiletine was not only blocking the sodium current that could benefit the patient, but the drug was also able to rescue the trafficking defect of the mutant, with a net effect of increasing the sustained current (LQT3 defect). Overall, the prevailing effect of mexiletine in this subject was the paradoxic worsening of the clinical phenotype.

In all, these studies demonstrate that the mutation-specific response to sodium channel blockers is related to identifiable biophysical properties of the channel, and prove the concept that in vitro analysis of the mutation can identify responders versus nonresponders and directly affect care decisions.

SUMMARY

Are we ready for genetic testing to be prime time? The answer is yes, depending on the condition: as is the case with any other medical testing, the ability of the care team involved to determine pretest probability of disease drives the appropriate usage of the technology. Overall, these observations highlight the concept that future research aimed at using genetic information for clinical and therapeutic management of patients with inherited arrhythmogenic disease might include the need of functional characterization, beyond DNA sequencing, to be able to provide tailored patient-specific health care. The authors support the view that the practical value of genetic analysis is different in the various inherited arrhythmogenic conditions; it is directly connected to the multidisciplinary approach whereby the cardiologist, the clinical geneticist, and the molecular biologist are coprotagonists of a medical action aimed to the best use of the genetic information. Genetic testing for inherited cardiac arrhythmias should not be the first test performed, but clearly has a prime-time place in current practice.

REFERENCES

1. Priori SG, Napolitano C. Role of genetic analyses in cardiology: part I: Mendelian diseases: cardiac channelopathies. Circulation 2006;113:1130–5.
2. Priori SG, Napolitano C. Genetics of long QT, Brugada and other channelopathies. In: Jalife J, Zipes DP, editors. Cardiac electrophysiology: from cell to bedside. 4th edition. Philadelphia: W.B. Saunders; 2004. p. 8.
3. Priori SG, Napolitano C, Vicentini A. Inherited arrhythmia syndromes: applying the molecular biology and genetics to the clinical management. J Interv Card Electrophysiol 2003;9:93–101.
4. Priori SG, Cantù F, Schwartz PJ. The long QT syndrome: new diagnostic and therapeutic approach in the era of molecular biology. Schweiz Med Wochenschr 1996;126:1727–31.
5. Viskin S, Rosovski U, Sands AJ, et al. Inaccurate electrocardiographic interpretation of long QT: the majority of physicians cannot recognize a long QT when they see one. Heart Rhythm 2005;2(6):569–74.
6. MacCormick JM, McAlister H, Crawford J, et al. Misdiagnosis of long QT syndrome as epilepsy at first presentation. Ann Emerg Med 2009;54(1):26–32.
7. Priori SG, Schwartz PJ, Napolitano C, et al. Risk stratification in the long-QT syndrome. N Engl J Med 2003;348:1866–74.
8. Mohler PJ, Schott JJ, Gramolini AO, et al. Ankyrin-B mutation causes type 4 long-QT cardiac arrhythmia and sudden cardiac death. Nature 2003;421(6923):634–9.
9. Sansone V, Tawil R. Management and treatment of Andersen-Tawil syndrome (ATS). Neurotherapeutics 2007;4:233–7.
10. Splawsky I, Timothy KW, Sharpe LM, et al. Ca(V)1.2 calcium channel dysfunction causes a multisystem disorder including arrhythmia and autism. Cell 2004;119(1):19–31.
11. Napolitano C, Priori SG, Schwartz PJ, et al. Genetic testing in the long QT syndrome: development and validation of an efficient approach to genotyping in clinical practice. JAMA 2005;294(23):2975–80.
12. Priori SG, Bloise R, Crotti L. The long QT syndrome. Europace 2001;3:16–27.
13. Schwartz PJ, Moss AJ, Vincent GM, et al. Diagnostic criteria for the long QT syndrome. An update. Circulation 1993;88(2):782–4.
14. Tester DJ, Will ML, Haglund CM, et al. Effect of clinical phenotype on yield of long QT syndrome genetic testing. J Am Coll Cardiol 2006;47(4):764–8.

15. Moss AJ, Zareba W, Benhorin J, et al. ECG T-wave patterns in genetically distinct forms of the hereditary long QT syndrome. Circulation 1995;92(10): 2929–34.

16. Zhang L, Timothy KW, Vincent GM, et al. Spectrum of ST-T-wave patterns and repolarization parameters in congenital long-QT syndrome: ECG findings identify genotypes. Circulation 2000;102(23):2849–55.

17. Schwartz PJ, Priori SG, Spazzolini C, et al. Genotype-phenotype correlation in the long-QT syndrome: gene-specific triggers for life-threatening arrhythmias. Circulation 2001;103(1):89–95.

18. Priori SG, Napolitano C, Schwartz PJ, et al. Association of long QT syndrome loci and cardiac events among patients treated with beta-blockers. JAMA 2004;292(11):1341–4.

19. Zareba W, Moss AJ, Schwartz PJ, et al. Influence of genotype on the clinical course of the long-QT syndrome. International long-QT syndrome registry research group. N Engl J Med 1998;339(14):960–5.

20. Moss AJ, Shimizu W, Wilde AA, et al. Clinical aspects of type-1 long-QT syndrome by location, coding type, and biophysical function of mutations involving the KCNQ1 gene. Circulation 2007; 115(19):2481–9.

21. Moss AJ, Zareba W, Hall WJ, et al. Effectiveness and limitations of beta-blocker therapy in congenital long-QT syndrome. Circulation 2000;101(6):616–23.

22. Moss AJ, Zareba W, Kaufman ES, et al. Increased risk of arrhythmic events in long-QT syndrome with mutations in the pore region of the human ether-a-go-go-related gene potassium channel. Circulation 2002;105:794–9.

23. Crotti L, Spazzolini C, Schwartz PJ, et al. The common long-QT syndrome mutation KCNQ1/A341V causes unusually severe clinical manifestations in patients with different ethnic backgrounds: toward a mutation-specific risk stratification. Circulation 2007;116(21):2366–75.

24. Liu JF, Goldenberg I, Moss AJ, et al. Phenotypic variability in Caucasian and Japanese patients with matched LQT1 mutations. Ann Noninvasive Electrocardiol 2008;13(3):234–41.

25. Brugada P, Brugada J. Right bundle branch block, persistent ST segment elevation and sudden cardiac death: a distinct clinical and electrocardiographic syndrome. A multicenter report. J Am Coll Cardiol 1992;20(6):1391–6.

26. Fowler SJ, Priori SG. Clinical spectrum of patients with a Brugada ECG. Curr Opin Cardiol 2009; 24(1):74–81.

27. Thomas K, Grant AO. Ethnicity and arrhythmia susceptibility. J Cardiovasc Electrophysiol 2008; 19(4):427–9.

28. Chen Q, Kirsch GE, Zhang D, et al. Genetic basis and molecular mechanism for idiopathic ventricular fibrillation. Nature 1998;392(6673):293–6.

29. Ruan Y, Liu N, Priori SG. Sodium channel mutations and arrhythmias. Nat Rev Cardiol 2009;6(5):337–48.

30. Antzelevitch C, Brugada P, Borggrefe M, et al. Brugada syndrome: report of the second consensus conference: endorsed by the heart rhythm society and the European Heart Rhythm Association. Circulation 2005;111(5):659–70.

31. Shimizu W, Aiba T, Kamakura S. Mechanisms of disease: current understanding and future challenges in Brugada syndrome. Nat Clin Pract Cardiovasc Med 2005;2(8):408–14.

32. Priori SG, Napolitano C, Gasparini M, et al. Natural history of Brugada syndrome: insights for risk stratification and management. Circulation 2002;105(11): 1342–7.

33. London B, Michalec M, Mehdi H, et al. Mutation in glycerol-3-phosphate dehydrogenase 1 like gene (GPD1-L) decreases cardiac Na^+ current and causes inherited arrhythmias. Circulation 2007; 116(20):2260–8.

34. Antzelevitch C, Pollevick GD, Cordeiro JM, et al. Loss-of-function mutations in the cardiac calcium channel underlie a new clinical entity characterized by ST-segment elevation, short QT intervals, and sudden cardiac death. Circulation 2007;115(4):442–9.

35. Watanabe H, Koopmann TT, Le Scouarnec S, et al. Sodium channel beta1 subunit mutations associated with Brugada syndrome and cardiac conduction disease in humans. J Clin Invest 2008;118(6):2260–8.

36. Delpon E, Cordeiro JM, Nunez L, et al. Functional effects of KCNE3 mutation and its role in the development of Brugada syndrome. Circ Arrhythm Electrophysiol 2008;1(3):209–18.

37. Hu D, Martinez HI, Burashnikov E, et al. A mutation in the b3 subunit of the cardiac sodium channel associated with Brugada ECG phenotype. Circ Cardiovasc Genet 2009;vol. 2(3):270–8.

38. Smits JP, Eckardt L, Probst V, et al. Genotype-phenotype relationship in Brugada syndrome: electrocardiographic features differentiate SCN5A-related patients from nonSCN5A-related patients. J Am Coll Cardiol 2002;40(2):350–6.

39. Bezzina CR, Shimizu W, Yang P, et al. Common sodium channel promoter haplotype in Asian subjects underlies variability in cardiac conduction. Circulation 2006;113(3):338–44.

40. Yamada T, Watanabe I, Okumura Y, et al. Atrial electrophysiological abnormality in patients with Brugada syndrome assessed by P-wave signal-averaged ECG and programmed atrial stimulation. Circ J 2006;70(12):1574–9.

41. Yokokawa M, Noda T, Okamura H, et al. Comparison of long-term follow-up of electrocardiographic features in Brugada syndrome between the SCN5A-positive probands and the SCN5A-negative probands. Am J Cardiol 2007;100(4): 649–55.

42. Rossenbacker T, Carroll SJ, Liu H, et al. Novel pore mutation in SCN5A manifests as a spectrum of phenotypes ranging from atrial flutter, conduction disease and Brugada syndrome to sudden cardiac death. Heart Rhythm 2004;1(5):610–5.

43. Kyndt F, Probst V, Potet F, et al. Novel SCN5A mutation leading either to isolated cardiac conduction defect or Brugada syndrome in a large French family. Circulation 2001;104(25):3081–6.

44. Schott JJ, Alshinawi C, Kyndt F, et al. Cardiac conduction defects associate with mutations in SCN5A. Nat Genet 1999;23(1):20–1.

45. Olson TM, Michels VV, Ballew JD, et al. Sodium channel mutations and susceptibility to heart failure and atrial fibrillation. JAMA 2005;293(4):447–54.

46. Frustaci A, Priori SG, Pieroni M, et al. Cardiac histological substrate in patients with clinical phenotype of Brugada syndrome. Circulation 2005;112(24): 3680–7.

47. Catalano O, Antonaci S, Moro G, et al. Magnetic resonance investigations in Brugada syndrome reveal unexpectedly high rate of structural abnormalities. Eur Heart J 2009;30(18):2241–8.

48. McNair WP, Ku L, Taylor MR, et al. SCN5A mutation associated with dilated cardiomyopathy, conduction disorder, and arrhythmia. Circulation 2004;110(15): 2163–7.

49. Cerrone M, Noujaim SF, Tolkacheva EG, et al. Arrhythmogenic mechanisms in a mouse model of catecholaminergic polymorphic ventricular tachycardia. Circ Res 2007;101(10):1039–48.

50. Priori SG, Napolitano C, Memmi M, et al. Clinical and molecular characterization of patients with catecholaminergic polymorphic ventricular tachycardia. Circulation 2002;106(1):69–74.

51. Napolitano C, Priori SG. Diagnosis and treatment of catecholaminergic polymorphic ventricular tachycardia. Heart Rhythm 2007;4(5):675–8.

52. Priori SG, Napolitano C, Tiso N, et al. Mutations in the cardiac ryanodine receptor gene (hRyR2) underlie catecholaminergic polymorphic ventricular tachycardia. Circulation 2001;103(2):196–200.

53. Lahat H, Pras E, Eldar M. RYR2 and CASQ2 mutations in patients suffering from catecholaminergic polymorphic ventricular tachycardia. Circulation 2003;107(3):e29; [author reply: e29].

54. Cerrone M, Colombi B, Bloise R, et al. Clinical and molecular characterization of a large cohort of patients affected with catecholaminergic polymorphic ventricular tachycardia. Circulation 2004;110 (Suppl II):2.

55. Tristani-Firouzi M, Jensen JL, Donaldson MR, et al. Functional and clinical characterization of KCNJ2 mutations associated with LQT7 (Andersen syndrome). J Clin Invest 2002;110:381–8.

56. Maron BJ, Gardin JM, Flack JM, et al. Prevalence of hypertrophic cardiomyopathy in a general

population of young adults. Echocardiographic analysis of 4111 subjects in the CARDIA study. Circulation 1995;92(4):785–9.

57. Van Dijk SJ, Dooijes D, dos Remedios C, et al. Cardiac myosin-binding protein C mutations and hypertrophic cardiomyopathy: haploinsufficiency, deranged phosphorylation, and cardiomyocyte dysfunction. Circulation 2009;119(11):1473–83.

58. Wigle ED, Ten Cate FJ, Spirito P, et al. American College of Cardiology/European Society of Cardiology clinical expert consensus document on hypertrophic cardiomyopathy. A report of the American College of Cardiology Foundation Task Force on clinical expert consensus documents and the European Society of Cardiology Committee for Practice Guidelines. J Am Coll Cardiol 2003;42(9):1687–713.

59. Leonardi S, Raineri C, De Ferrari GM, et al. Usefulness of cardiac magnetic resonance in assessing the risk of ventricular arrhythmias and sudden death in patients with hypertrophic cardiomyopathy. Eur Heart J 2009;30(16):2003–10.

60. Keren A, Syrris P, McKenna WJ. Hypertrophic cardiomyopathy: the genetic determinants of clinical disease expression. Nat Clin Pract Cardiovasc Med 2008;5(3):158–68.

61. Perkins MJ, Van Driest SL, Ellsworth EG, et al. Gene-specific modifying effects of pro-LVH polymorphisms involving the renin-angiotensin-aldosterone system among 389 unrelated patients with hypertrophic cardiomyopathy. Eur Heart J 2005;26(22): 2457–62.

62. Coats CJ, Elliott PM. Current management of hypertrophic cardiomyopathy. Curr Treat Options Cardiovasc Med 2008;10(6):496–504.

63. Marian AJ. Genetic determinants of cardiac hypertrophy. Curr Opin Cardiol 2008;23(3):199–205.

64. Watkins H, Rosenzweig A, Hwang DS, et al. Characteristics and prognostic implications of myosin missense mutations in familial hypertrophic cardiomyopathy. N Engl J Med 1992;326(17): 1108–14.

65. Charron P, Dubourg O, Desnos M, et al. Genotype-phenotype correlations in familial hypertrophic cardiomyopathy. A comparison between mutations in the cardiac protein-C and the beta-myosin heavy chain genes. Eur Heart J 1998;19(1):139–45.

66. Hershberger RE, Lindenfeld J, Mestroni L, et al. Genetic evaluation of cardiomyopathy—a Heart Failure Society of America practice guideline. J Card Fail 2009;15(2):83–97.

67. Watkins H, Ashrafian H, McKenna WJ. The genetics of hypertrophic cardiomyopathy: Teare redux. Heart 2008;94(10):1264–8.

68. Awad MM, Calkins H, Judge DP. Mechanisms of disease: molecular genetics of arrhythmogenic right ventricular dysplasia/cardiomyopathy. Nat Clin Pract Cardiovasc Med 2008;5(5):258–67.

69. Sen-Chowdhry S, McKenna WJ. Sudden cardiac death in the young: a strategy for prevention by targeted evaluation. Cardiology 2006;105(4):196–206.

70. Coonar AS, Protonotarios N, Tsatsopoulou A, et al. Gene for arrhythmogenic right ventricular cardiomyopathy with diffuse nonepidermolytic palmoplantar keratoderma and woolly hair (Naxos disease) maps to 17q21. Circulation 1998;97(20):2049–58.

71. Syrris P, Ward D, Asimaki A, et al. Desmoglein-2 mutations in arrhythmogenic right ventricular cardiomyopathy: a genotype-phenotype characterization of familial disease. Eur Heart J 2007;28(5):581–8.

72. Asimaki A, Tandri H, Huang H, et al. A new diagnostic test for arrhythmogenic right ventricular cardiomyopathy. N Engl J Med 2009;360(11):1075–84.

73. Sen-Chowdhry S, Syrris P, McKenna WJ. Role of genetic analysis in the management of patients with arrhythmogenic right ventricular dysplasia/cardiomyopathy. J Am Coll Cardiol 2007;50(19):1813–21.

74. Dalal D, Molin LH, Piccini J, et al. Clinical features of arrhythmogenic right ventricular dysplasia/cardiomyopathy associated with mutations in plakophilin-2. Circulation 2006;113(13):1641–9.

75. Calkins H, Marcus F. Arrhythmogenic right ventricular cardiomyopathy/dysplasia: an update. Curr Cardiol Rep 2008;10(5):367–75.

76. Harper PS. Practical genetic counselling. 5th edition. London: Wright; 1998.

77. Van der Roest WP, Pennings JM, Bakker M, et al. Family letters are an effective way to inform relatives about inherited cardiac disease. Am J Med Genet A 2009;149A(3):357–63.

78. Bai R, Napolitano C, Bloise R, et al. Yield of genetic screening in inherited cardiac channelopathies: how to prioritize access to genetic testing. Circ Arrhythm Electrophysiol 2009;2:6–15.

79. Priori SG, Napolitano C, Schwartz PJ, et al. The elusive link between LQT3 and Brugada syndrome: the role of flecainide challenge. Circulation 2000;102(9):945–7.

80. Shimizu W, Antzelevitch C. Sodium channel block with mexiletine is effective in reducing dispersion of repolarization and preventing torsade des pointes in LQT2 and LQT3 models of the long-QT syndrome. Circulation 1997;96(6):2038–47.

81. Ruan Y, Liu N, Bloise R, et al. Gating properties of SCN5A mutations and the response to mexiletine in long-QT syndrome type 3 patients. Circulation 2007;116(10):1137–44.

Genetics for the Electrophysiologist: Take Home Messages for the Clinician

Carlo Napolitano, MD, PhD[a,b,*], Samori Cummings, MD[b]

KEYWORDS
- Cardiomyopathy • Genetics • Arrhythmias
- Potassium currents

GENES AND MECHANISMS OF ABNORMAL ELECTROCARDIOGRAMS IN THE STRUCTURALLY NORMAL HEART
Potassium Currents

Potassium currents are active in all phases of cardiac action potential but are mainly involved in the genesis of phase 1, phase 3, and resting membrane potential (phase 4). Genetic abnormalities of proteins conducting potassium currents are found in several patients with a spectrum of clinical phenotypes: long QT syndrome (LQTS), short QT syndrome (SQTS), familial atrial fibrillation (FAF), and Brugada syndrome (BrS).

KCNQ1

Mutations in the *KCNQ1* gene that encodes for the alpha subunit of the slow component of delayed rectifier (IKs) current (KVLQT1 or Kv7.1) are associated with the LQT1 variant of LQTS with a loss-of-function effect and SQTS type 2 (SQTS2)[1] or FAF[2] when they cause gain of function. Thus, the coexistence of the phenotypes of SQTS2 and FAF should always be considered in the clinical evaluation. Although SQTS type 1 (SQTS1) is rare, LQT1 accounts for 40% to 50% of patients with LQTS.[3,4]

IKs current plays an important role during phase 3 of the action potential and is specifically sensitive to catecholamine activation. Thus, *KCNQ1* mutations become more evident during increased sympathetic tone (exercise, acute emotions) when impaired IKs activation leads to a failure to shorten action potential (ie, QT interval). This mechanism can also explain the increased risk of cardiac events during exercise for patients with LQT1.[5] Altered response to sympathetic stimulation has also been associated with a mutation in a *KCNQ1*-interacting protein. A missense mutation of *AKAP9* (also called Yotiao or LQT11) has been reported in a single family.[6] This mutation disrupts the cAMP-mediated phosphorylation and catecholamine-dependent channel activation; thus it is pathophysiologically similar to LQT1.

KCNH2

KCNH2 encodes for the alpha subunit of the rapid component of the delayed rectifier (*hERG*,) channel, which participates in the control of cardiac repolarization, mainly during phase 3. *KCNH2* is associated with LQT2 and SQTS1. LQT2 is the second most common variant of LQTS (20%–30% of patients) and follows from the loss-of-function mutations. SQTS1 is caused by gain-of-function mutations and is an infrequent finding in the clinical setting. Only 3 *KCNH2* mutations linked to SQTS1 have been reported so far.

KCNJ2

Andersen-Tawil syndrome (also called LQT7) is caused by mutations in the *KCNJ2* gene encoding

[a] Molecular Cardiology Laboratories, IRCCS Fondazione Salvatore Maugeri, Via Maugeri 10, 27100, Pavia, Italy
[b] Cadiovascular Genetics, Leon Charney Division of Cardiology, New York University Medical Center, 403 East 34th Street, RIV 4th Floor, New York, NY 10016, USA
* Corresponding author. Molecular Cardiology, Fondazione Salvatore Maugeri, Via Maugeri 10, 27100, Pavia, Italy.
E-mail address: carlo.napolitan@nyumc.org

Card Electrophysiol Clin 2 (2010) 623–634
doi:10.1016/j.ccep.2010.09.009
1877-9182/10/$ — see front matter © 2010 Published by Elsevier Inc.

for the cardiac inward rectifier (IK1). IK1-conducting channel (Kir2.1) participates in the control of the late repolarization phase and resting membrane potential. LQT7 is a rare variant (approximately 1%), which can include, with some exceptions, extracardiac manifestations, such as typically periodic paralysis and dysmorphic features. The electrocardiogram (ECG) in those with LQT7 is characterized by giant U waves and frequent ventricular arrhythmias (often unrelated to adrenergic tone), including bidirectional tachycardia. Some patients with *KCNJ2* mutations may present a phenotype similar to that of catecholaminergic polymorphic ventricular tachycardia (CPVT), which is discussed later.

Potassium channel beta subunits

Additional potassium-related LQTS variants are those caused by mutations in the beta subunits *KCNE1-LQT5* (which co-assembles with *KCNQ1*) and *KCNE2-LQT6*, which are thought to coassemble mainly with *KCNH2* (but also with other potassium channels). These 2 genes cause LQT5 and LQT6, which together account for approximately 5% to 6% of cases. LQT5 and LQT6 have similar pathogenesis (and clinical presentation) as LQT1

and LQT2 but with a generally milder phenotype and lower penetrance.[3,7] A potassium channel beta subunit can also cause the BrS6 variant of BrS (**Table 1**). BrS6 was identified in a single family with a mutation of *KCNE3* gene encoding for the MiRP2 potassium channel beta subunit. When the mutated *KCNE3* was coexpressed in Chinese hamster ovary cells with Kv4.3 (the alpha subunit of the ion channel conducting the transient outward channel [Ito] current), an increase in the Ito current as well as an accelerated inactivation was observed.[8] BrS6 is probably rare and is not routinely screened at present.

Sodium Current

The cardiac sodium current (INa) controls fast depolarization (phase 0) of action potential. *SCN5A* is the gene that encodes for the INa-conducting protein NaV1.5. *SCN5A* mutations were first identified in the LQT3 variant of LQTS; in vitro expression demonstrated that these mutations result from a gain-of-function effect. This effect is typically because of an increased late INa but may also derive from a variety of kinetic abnormalities (shift of steady state inactivation

---

Table 1
Potassium currents in inherited arrhythmias

Current	Clinical Phenotype	Variant	Gene	Protein	Functional Abnormality
IKs	LQTS	LQT1	*KCNQ1*	Alpha subunit of IKs	↓
		LQT5	*KCNE1*	Slow delayed rectifier beta subunit	↓
		LQT11	*AKAP9*	Yotiao-Iks interacting protein	↓
	Atrial fibrillation	ATFB3	*KCNQ1*	Slow delayed rectifier alpha subunit	↑
	SQTS	SQTS2	*KCNQ1*	Slow delayed rectifier alpha subunit	↑
IKr	LQTS	LQTS2	*KCNH2*	Rapid delayed rectifier alpha subunit	↓
		LQT6	*KCNE2*	Rapid delayed rectifier beta subunit[a]	↓
	SQTS	SQT1	*KCNH2*	Rapid delayed rectifier alpha subunit	↑
IK1	Andersen-Tawil syndrome[b]	LQT7	*KCNJ2*	Inward rectifier alpha subunit	↓
	SQTS	SQTS3	*KCNJ2*	Inward rectifier alpha subunit	↑
Ito	BrS	BrS6	*KCNE3*	Transient outward current beta subunit	↑

Abbreviations: IKr, rapid component of the delayed rectifier; Ito, transient outward channel; ↓, loss of function; ↑, gain of function.
  [a] Some investigators suggested that MiRP can coassemble with multiple ion channels.
  [b] Cases of isolated QT prolongation without muscular involvement are reported. In other cases, phenocopy of CPVT may be observed.

and activation, increased window current, faster recovery from inactivation). Patients with LQT3 have an increased risk of events at rest or during sleep. SCN5A is not the only gene that can affect INa. LQT3-like phenotype can be seldom caused by mutations in the NaV1.5 accessory proteins, caveolin 3 (CAV3, LQT9),[9] sodium beta-4 subunit (SCN4B, LQT10), and syntrophin gene (SNTA1, LQT12).[10] In agreement with a common pathophysiology, mutations in these genes lead to a gain of function of INa. Independently from the causative gene, sodium-dependent LQTS is caused by an excess of depolarizing current with a consequent prolongation of the action potential.

SCN5A is also the most represented gene (15%–25%) among patients with BrS1. At variance with LQT3, BrS1 mutations cause a loss of function. Therefore, less sodium flows into the cell during depolarization. As in the case of LQT3, additional proteins affecting INa have been linked to BrS, such as GPD1-L, SCN1B, and SCNB3 (Table 2). GPD1-L (glycerol phosphate dehydrogenase) interacts with NaV1.5 channel, and when mutated, it causes reduced INa,[11] not very much dissimilar form the primary pore-forming channel mutations. GPD1-L mutations are infrequent among patients with BrS (1%–2%). SCN1B that encodes for the NaV1.5 beta-1 subunit is the cause of BrS7. Mutations in SCN1B were recently found to be associated with BrS in 3 European kindred[12] and to cause a loss of channel function. BrS5 genes have been recently identified in a single patient harboring a missense mutation of the SCN3B

gene.[13] This gene encodes for the beta-3 subunit of the cardiac sodium channel. SCNB3 influences the function of Nav1.5 mainly by controlling the intracellular trafficking of the channel. Accordingly, the mutation was found to result in reduced number of proteins correctly placed on the membrane and reduced current.

In some instances besides causing increased or reduced net INa, SCN5A mutations profoundly alter channel kinetic and voltage dependency. Such complexity of biophysical abnormalities may translate into clinical entities presenting at the same time features of BrS and LQTS, the so-called overlapping phenotypes.[14] The clinical presentation may include different combinations of ST elevation, prolonged QT interval, progressive conduction defect, and sinus node dysfunction. Therefore, clinical evaluation should consider the possibility of finding some features of BrS (such as conduction defect) in patients with LQT3 and vice versa. Some SCN5A mutations have been reported in association with sinus node dysfunction and dilated cardiomyopathy.

Calcium Current

L-type calcium channels become activated during phase 0 to 2 (plateau) of the action potential to generate the calcium current (ICa). The protein that conducts ICa is CaV1.2, which is encoded by the CACNA1c gene.

As it happens for most cardiac ion channel genes, mutations affecting CaV1.2 can bear a loss as well as a gain of function (Table 3). The

Table 2
Sodium current in inherited arrhythmias

Current	Clinical Phenotype	Variant	Gene	Protein	Functional Abnormality
INa	LQTS	LQT3	SCN5A	Sodium channel alpha subunit	↑
		LQT9	CAV3	Caveolin	↑
		LQT10	SCN4B	Sodium channel beta-4 subunit	↑
		LQT12	SNTA1	Syntrophin	↑
	BrS	BrS1	SCN5A	Sodium channel alpha subunit	↓
		BrS2	GPD1-L	Glycerol phosphate dehydrogenase	↓
		BrS5	SCN1B	Sodium channel beta-1 subunit	↓
		BrS7	SCNB3	Sodium channel beta-1 subunit	↓

Abbreviations: ↓, loss of function; ↑, gain of function.

Table 3
Inherited arrhythmias associated with calcium handling abnormalities

Current	Clinical Phenotype	Variant	Gene	Protein	Functional Abnormality
ICa	Timothy syndrome	TS1	*CACNA1c*	Calcium channel alpha subunit	↑
	BrS	BrS3	*CACNA1c*	Calcium channel alpha subunit	↓
		BrS4	*CACNB2*	Calcium channel beta subunit	↓
SR calcium release	Catecholaminergic polymorphic ventricular tachycardia	CPVT1	*RyR2*	SR calcium releasing channel	Calcium overload
	Catecholaminergic polymorphic ventricular tachycardia	CPVT1	*CASQ2*	Calsequestrin	Calcium overload

Abbreviations: SR, sarcoplasmic reticulum; ↓, loss of function; ↑, gain of function.

first *CACNA1c* mutation was reported by the authors' group in a collaborative study with Splawski and colleagues.[15] In this study, the investigators described the association of this gene with Timothy syndrome (also called LQT8). This LQTS variant presents an extremely severe and rare phenotype, including QT prolongation, atrioventricular block, syndactyly, congenital heart defects, autism, reduced immune response, and developmental disorders.[15] Very few patients with Timothy syndrome have survived after puberty in the reported series.[16] In vitro expression of the mutation responsible for Timothy syndrome showed a loss of voltage dependency of the channels that fail to inactivate with a consequent gain-of-function effect. All the cases of Timothy syndrome reported so far have only 2 different mutations. Thus, the genetic testing for this variant is quick and has high success rate.[17]

Cardiac calcium channel abnormalities have been also reported in few patients with BrS also presenting with a short corrected QT interval (QTc, <360 millisecond).[18] Two genes encoding for calcium channel constitutive proteins have been involved, mutant *CACNA1c* (the same as that of LQT8), causing BrS3, was found in 2 of a series of 82 patients, whereas *CACNB2*, causing BrS4, was found in 1 patient from the same cohort. *CACNA1c* and *CACNB2* constitute the alpha and beta subunits of the cardiac voltage-dependent calcium channel, respectively, and in both cases, the mutations of these genes cause a loss of function with reduced calcium entry and shortening of the phase 2 of action potential.

Intracellular Calcium Handling Disease

The pivotal role of calcium(Ca^{2+}) ion handling for the maintenance of the physiologic properties of the heart is highlighted by the evidence that cellular Ca^{2+} fluxes are found in several diseases, such as heart failure, cardiac hypertrophy, and inherited arrhythmias.[19,20] There are several important players of intracellular calcium handling, but so far only 2 have been associated with inherited arrhythmogenic disorders, namely, the ryanodine receptor (RyR2) and the cardiac calsequestrin (calsequestrin 2 gene [*CASQ2*]). Mutations in both genes are associated with a severe phenotype, the CPVT. CPVT manifests with adrenergic-dependent arrhythmias and sudden death in the setting of an unremarkable resting ECG but a typical pattern of bidirectional or polymorphic ventricular tachycardia that can be reproducibly elicited during exercise or catecholamine infusion.

Two genetic variants of CPVT have been identified by linkage analysis and candidate gene screening, CPVT1 with autosomal dominant transmission and CPVT2 with autosomal recessive transmission. CPVT1 is largely more prevalent (approximately 50% of patients); it is caused by mutations in the RyR2 gene, encoding for the cardiac ryanodine receptor, that were initially reported in 2001 by Priori and colleagues.[21] The ryanodine receptor is a tetrameric Ca^{2+} release channel spanning the membrane of the sarcoplasmic reticulum (SR) and is required for excitation-contraction coupling. During phase 2 of action potential, the Ca^{2+} entry through the voltage-gated plasmalemmal L-type calcium channels triggers the opening of RyR2 (which are located at T tubules in close proximity with the calcium channels), and a large amount of Ca^{2+} from the SR enters the cytoplasm and is made available for contraction (the so-called calcium-induced calcium release process). Approximately 140 *RyR2* mutations have been reported, and these mutations tend to affect specific clusters or regions of the protein.[22] Despite the proposal of multiple biophysical mechanisms, the final common pathway of CPVT mutations is a Ca^{2+} leakage from the SR to cytosol. The Ca^{2+} overload activates the sodium-calcium exchanger and the development of delayed afterdepolarization (DAD).[23] During adrenergic activation, Ca^{2+} leak is exacerbated (mainly by an increase of SR calcium content) and DADs may reach the threshold to generate spontaneous action potentials (the so-called triggered activity).[23]

The autosomal recessive variant, CPVT2, is caused by mutations of *CASQ2*.[24] Data from the authors' CPVT registry suggest that *CASQ2* mutations account for 3% to 5% of all genotyped patients.[25] Calsequestrin is a calcium-buffering protein primarily expressed in the terminal cisternae of the SR. Mutant *CASQ2* loses the buffering capacity and polymerization properties and also directly affects RyR2 function by increasing its open probability.[26] It has also been demonstrated in CPVT2 animal models that *CASQ2* induces a dramatic reduction of the protein level.[27,28]

More recently it has been proposed that mutations of two other genes may cause an arrhythmogenic disorder that resembles the classical description of CPVT (phenocopies; see **Table 3**). *KCNJ2*, which is more frequently associated with Andersen syndrome (LQT7), may cause bidirectional VT with mild or absent QT prolongation and no extracardiac involvement. Anecdotal reports show that *ANK2* (gene for LQT4) mutations may cause a CPVT phenotype.[29] Although there is no systematic assessment of the relative prevalence of this variant, it is probably rare, and there is no current indication for a systematic screening of this gene in patients with CPVT.

GENES AND MECHANISMS OF ARRHYTHMOGENIC STRUCTURAL CARDIOMYOPATHIES

Two forms of inherited cardiomyopathy, arrhythmogenic right ventricular cardiomyopathy (ARVC) or dysplasia and hypertrophic cardiomyopathy (HCM), are relevant to clinical electrophysiologists because these cardiomyopathies primarily manifest with cardiac arrhythmias and increased risk of sudden cardiac death. The distinction between these two disorders is not only possible on a clinical base but also from a genetic standpoint; ARVC is now considered a disease of the desmosome and cell-to-cell junction, whereas HCM is mainly caused by a dysfunction of the contractile elements of the myocardial cells.

Desmosomal Disease

When cell-to-cell connecting structure is sick, the myocardial wall becomes less resistant to tension and mechanical stress. This condition is the major abnormality underlying ARVC, which is a disorder of the cardiac desmosome, a macromolecular complex responsible for supporting structural stability through cell-cell adhesion. Desmosomes also have other functions that may participate in ARVC pathophysiology, such as gene transcriptional control (mostly genes of adipogenesis and apoptotic cascade), electrical conductivity (through regulation of gap junctions), and calcium homeostasis.[30]

There are currently 6 known genes (**Table 4**), 5 encoding for constitutive desmosomal proteins and 1 encoding for growth factor. According to the recent literature,[30,31] *PKP2* (plakophilin-2 gene) encoding for a desmosomal protein is the most frequently detected cause of ARVC and encompasses 20% to 40% of cases. Desmoglein (*DSG2*) accounts for 15% to 30% of cases, followed by desmoplakin (*DSP*), which accounts for 5% to 15% of cases. Plakoglobin (*JUP*) and desmocollin (*DSC2*) are rare causes of ARVC. In addition, several ARVC chromosomal loci (regions where a disease-causing gene may be located) have been identified, but the corresponding gene is still unknown.[30] On the basis of the available data, the molecular pathogenesis of ARVC is that of a mutation-dependent impaired mechanical coupling or desmosome disruption, followed by apoptosis and fatty degeneration with remodeling of the intercalated discs. The preferential right ventricular localization of ARVC is explained with the natural lower tolerance of the right ventricle to wall tension. This reason also explains why ARVC is primarily an arrhythmogenic condition; the lack of involvement of left ventricle preserves hemodynamic function. Progressive degeneration of areas in the right ventricle (typical from epicardium toward endocardium) creates inhomogeneous conduction and the substrate for reentry. Patients often present with palpitations, syncope, and sometimes cardiac arrest (typically triggered by exercise) before overt right ventricular abnormalities become detectable. In rare instances,

Table 4
Desmosomal and sarcomeric protein in inherited arrhythmias with structural involvement

Locus Name	Gene Symbol	Phenotype	Protein	Estimated Prevalence (%)
CMH1	MYH7	HCM	β-myosin heavy chain	35–45
CMH2	TNNT2	HCM	Cardiac troponin T	5–10
CMH3	TPM1	HCM	α-tropomyosin	1–5
CMH4	MYBPC3	HCM	Cardiac myosin binding protein C	20–50
CMH7	TNNI3	HCM	Cardiac troponin I	1–5
CMH8	MYL3	HCM	Cardiac essential myosin light chain	1–51
CMH9	TTN	HCM	Titin	<1
CMH10	MYL2	HCM	Cardiac regulatory myosin light chain	<1
CMH11	ACTC	HCM	Actin	<1
CMH13	TNNC1	HCM	Cardiac troponin C	0.4
CMH14	MYH6	HCM	α-myosin heavy chain	<1
ARVC1	TGFB3	ARVC	Transforming factor β subunit	<1
ARVC8	DSP	ARVC	Desmoplakin	5–15
ARVC9	PKP2	ARVC	Plakophilin	20–40
ARVC10	DSG2	ARVC	Desmoglein	12–40
ARVC11	DSC2	ARVC	Desmocollin	<1
ARVC12	JUP	ARVC	Plakoglobin	<1

ARVC can involve the left ventricle and progress to heart failure.[31] Rare cases of ARVC caused by a nondesmosomal protein are possible. In this case, the TGFβ3[32] protein stimulates mesenchymal cells to proliferate and to produce extracellular matrix components. TGFβ3 induces a fibrotic response in various tissues in vivo. Thus, mutations of TGFβ3 gene could promote myocardial fibrosis and disrupt electrical and mechanical behavior.

Sarcomere Disease

An altered function of proteins of the cardiac sarcomere is the most frequent and typical cause of HCM. In such instances, myocardial hypertrophy is the only phenotype (pure HCM; see **Table 4**). Nonsarcomeric proteins have also been associated with HCM in a minority of cases. These variants usually show additional phenotypes such as abnormal conduction pathways (Wolff-Parkinson-White syndrome), sensorineural deafness, neurologic and neurogenic muscular atrophy, trunk hypotonia, and encephalopathy.[30]

HCM is a disorder of contractile function. In this context, hypertrophy represents an adaptation to the inability to generate sufficient strength to maintain adequate cardiac output. Fibroblast proliferation (fibrosis) and tissue disarray are the result of such adaptive modifications. Functional expression studies of mutant sarcomeric proteins show a variety of abnormalities, spanning defects in myofibril formation, altered ATPase activity, Ca^{2+} sensitivity, and impaired actin-myosin interaction.

Most cases of HCM are transmitted as an autosomal dominant trait, whereas other uncommon variants are inherited as autosomal, recessive, X-linked, or mitochondrial disorders. At present, 24 genes encoding various sarcomeric, calcium handling, and mitochondrial proteins have been identified. Mutations in the HCM genes may have extremely late manifestations and cause mild forms of ventricular hypertrophy in the elderly, which were often considered as acquired conditions.[33] The prevalence of HCM is estimated to be 1 in 500, making HCM one of the most prevalent genetic diseases. HCM is characterized by a wide spectrum of clinical phenotypes with incomplete and time-dependent penetrance. The molecular epidemiology of HCM has been systematically addressed[34] by screening the entire open reading frame of 9 HCM genes in 197 probands (MYH7, MYBPC3, TNNI3, TNNT2, MYL2, MYL3,

TPM1, ACTC, TNNC1). Approximately 63% of these patients have been successfully genotyped. Two genes, *MYH7* and *MYBPC3*, were present in 82% of genotyped patients, whereas troponin T and troponin I were present in 6.5% of probands. Therefore, a genetic screening limited to the 4 major genes leads to the identification of the genetic defect in more that 90% of patients with clinically confirmed HCM.

Fibrosis and disarray create the substrate for reentry arrhythmias, which constitute the primary manifestation of HCM. In several cases, sudden death may be the first manifestation of the disease.[35] At later stage, hemodynamic dysfunction can occur with progression to heart failure. HCM is diagnosed when left ventricular hypertrophy (typically asymmetric in distribution) is evident in the absence of cardiac or systemic conditions (eg, hypertension or aortic stenosis) that could potentially induce hypertrophy of the magnitude observed.

THE USE OF GENETICS IN THE CLINICAL SETTING

Genetic tests are progressively entering the clinical practice and are applied not only for genetic conditions but also for risk stratification in multifactorial disorders that may have a genetic predisposition[36,37] or to assess response to drugs.[38] The field of inherited arrhythmogenic diseases is not an exception. Therefore, it becomes important that genetic testing is used in a correct way to not lose potential benefits and also to not stretch the indications. Performing genetic analysis without clear clinical indications and endpoints may bring about more problems than solutions.

Genetic Testing and Clinical Diagnosis

Genetic testing is primarily indicated when clinical diagnosis is certain. In such instances, genetic testing may provide a spectrum of clinically useful information, such as reproductive and familial risk assessment, preventive therapies, risk stratification, and therapeutic choice selection. On the other hand, as already reported,[17] it is important to consider that the applicability of genetic testing is variable according to the underlying disease, and the applicability spans from simple diagnosis confirmation and reproductive risk detection (eg, as in ARVC) to consistent genotype-based risk stratification and therapy as in LQTS.[7,39]

When a mutation is eventually identified in clinically affected probands, screening of all family members becomes indicated. First- and second-degree relatives should undergo clinical and genetic evaluation whenever possible; genetic

testing should also be performed in individuals with negative phenotype. With this approach it is possible to assess cosegregation (concordance between genotype and phenotype) that may be of substantial help when mutations of uncertain meaning are identified; furthermore, the identification of nonpenetrant carriers allows the prevention of potential triggers for cardiac events (eg, QT-prolonging drugs in LQTS or fever in BrS)[40,41] and administration of therapy for primary prevention, when indicated (eg, in LQTS and CPVT).[42]

Genetic Testing in Borderline Cases

It is often tempting to use genetic screening as a tool to reach a diagnosis when clinical evaluation is inconclusive. In some cases, the report of the diagnostic laboratory provides the required answer if a known pathogenetic mutation is identified. However, it is important to be aware that in such instances (ie, when clinical diagnosis is uncertain), the probability of identification of a genetic defect is significantly reduced. The authors quantified the yield of genetic screening of LQTS, BrS, and CPVT genes based on entry criteria and observed a sharp decrease in the success rate according to the level of confidence of clinical diagnosis. The percentage of identified mutations was reduced from 64% to 14% and from 62% to 5% in the presence of a conclusive or a possible diagnosis in patients with LQTS and CPVT, respectively. This result suggests that (1) the use of a genetic testing to confirm or dismiss the diagnosis in borderline cases has a high rate of negative results, (2) communication with the patients should not place too much emphasis and expectations on the test, and (3) the cost-effectiveness (cost per identified mutation) of genetic testing is poor when diagnosis is uncertain.

The Role of Functional Characterization of Mutants

Even once a genetic variant is identified, the association with the clinical presentation might not be straightforward. The pathogenetic role of novel (not published) single amino acid substitutions, especially when present in families with incomplete penetrance, may be difficult to be established. Further analysis of location, phylogenetic conservation, and ethnic-specific variants can support the interpretation process.[43] In other instances, the role of identified variants remains blurred. Therefore, it becomes rational to use in vitro expression of mutants. Although in vitro functional characterization is not widely available and soars the genotyping bill, there are indications that the technique may provide useful information.

Moss and colleagues[44] have shown that KCNQ1 (LQT1) mutations causing a dominant negative effect in vitro are associated with a worse outcome and 2.2-fold risk increase events. In other cases, in vitro expression provides therapeutic indications. In 2000, Benhorin and colleagues[45] provided in vitro and clinical evidence that the QTc shortens in carriers of D1790 G when they receive flecainide but not when they are treated with lidocaine. The authors further extended this observation by analyzing a series of SCN5A mutations associated with differential response to mexiletine treatment.[46] After performing a systematic characterization of the mutant channels, the authors were able to propose that a hyperpolarizing shift of inactivation is associated with a good clinical response to mexiletine (**Fig. 1**). Along the same line, it was also demonstrated that in vitro expression might find an explanation of the paradoxic effects (worsening of phenotype) of mexiletine.[47]

Genotyping of Common Variants and Clinical Management

An interesting and promising area of research, which is going to represent an important source of information to link the genetic substrate with the clinics (thus leading to improved risk stratification and clinical management), derives from the evidence of variable expressivity and incomplete penetrance in these disorders. Differential severity of clinical phenotypes is frequently observed not only in patients with mutation on the same gene but also among those who harbor exactly the same mutation. Thus, the identification of modifier genes is an attractive possibility for the improvement of genotype-based risk stratification. Genetic modifiers are represented by frequent genetic variants in the population that per se are neither sufficient nor necessary to cause the disease but can worsen or attenuate the phenotype.

Multiple Mutants as Modifiers

The evidence of multiple mutations on disease-causing genes was the first, and rather

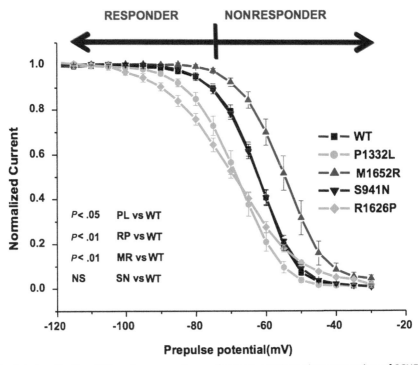

Fig. 1. Steady state inactivation (SSI) and response to mexiletine in LQT3. In vitro expression of SCN5A mutants in LQT3 predicts clinical efficacy of mexiletine. The SSI kinetics of 4 NaV1.5 mutations is depicted. The mutations that cause a negative shift of SSI (*green lines*) are associated with clinically relevant QTc shortening and lack of events at follow-up. Neutral or positive SSI shift is characterized by poor response. WT, wild type. Different SCN5A mutations: MR, M1652R; PL, P1332L; RP, R1626P; SN, S941N. (*From* Ruan Y, Liu N, Bloise R, et al. Gating properties of SCN5A mutations and the response to mexiletine in long-QT syndrome type 3 patients. Circulation 2007;116:1140; with permission.)

straightforward, hypothesis raised by several investigators to account for phenotype variability. The hypothesis is based on the evidence that a nontrivial percentage of patients with inherited arrhythmogenic conditions present more than one mutation. Double mutations are present in 5% to 8% of patients with LQTS,[3,43] in 3% to 5% of those with HCM,[48,49] and in 3.5% to 7% of those with ARVC.[50] In 2004, Westenskow and colleagues[51] were the first to report that LQTS-associated compound mutations cause a severe phenotype, whereas Kobori and colleagues[52] suggested that these mutations may reduce the response to β-blockers. However, although pathophysiologically sound and supported by preliminary evidence, a systematic assessment of specific features of carriers of double mutations has never been performed because of the lack of large cohorts. Therefore, there is no quantitative figure of the associated risk and prognosis.

Genetic Modifiers of Electrical Substrate

Dissecting the heritable nature of the ECG and the common genetic factors, which may predispose to cardiac arrhythmias in the population, has become a primary goal of genetic research in cardiology. Several candidate gene or genome-wide association studies has allowed to draw a list of single nucleotide polymorphisms (SNPs) that modify QT interval,[53,54] QRS duration,[55] and heart rate[56,57] in the healthy population. The use of this information to detect genetic modifiers in inherited arrhythmia syndromes directly follows this line of research.

Initial reports focused on the role of common variants in the same disease-causing genes, such as the SCN5A-H558R and the KCNH2-K897 T, in modulating the clinical expression of primary mutations.[58–60] Some investigators have reported that the effect of such common SNPs may be mutation specific. For example, the loss-of-function (Brugada-like) defect D1275 N in SCN5A was rescued by R558 through enhancing cell surface targeting. In contrast, the defects of mutants E161 K, P1298 L, and R1632H were aggravated in the R558 background.[60] Functional SNP mutation interaction has also been reported for the KCNH2-K897 T, which also has a QT modulatory effect on large series of healthy subjects.[61]

Overall, these data suggest a role of SNP as modifiers in anecdotal cases but are far from bringing about implications for population-wise risk stratification. This latter issue has been investigated in only few studies focusing on NOS1AP gene, which has the strongest QT modulatory effect in the general population.[54] NOS1AP is involved in nitric oxide production and action potential duration modulation via an effect on

	LQT1 Males	LQT1 Females	LQT2/3 Males	LQT2/3 Females
QTc ≥500 ms rs366 minor	4.08	6.24	7.18	10.97
QTc ≥500 ms rs366 common	2.78	4.25	4.89	7.47
QTc <500 ms rs366 minor	1.47	2.24	2.58	3.95
QTc <500 ms rs366 common	1	1.53	1.76	2.69

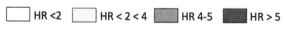

☐ HR <2   ☐ HR < 2 < 4   ▨ HR 4–5   ■ HR > 5

Fig. 2. LQTS risk stratification scheme. NOS1AP improves genotype-based risk stratification in LQTS. Each box shows the hazard ratio (HR) for patients with different clinical and genetic profile. An HR of 1 with the following characteristics is the reference category: LQT1, male gender, QTc less than 500 millisecond, and homozygous for the common allele of NOS1AP rs10494366 (allele "TT" is abbreviated as rs366). (*From* Tomas M, Napolitano C, De Giuli L, et al. Polymorphisms in the NOS1AP gene modulate QT interval duration and risk of arrhythmias in the long QT Syndrome. J Am Coll Cardiol 2010;(55)24:2750; with permission.)

Ca^{2+} and potassium ion currents.[62] A recent study limited to an ethnically isolated population carrier of a single *KCNQ1* mutation (A341 V) suggested that *NOS1AP* influences QT duration in LQTS.[63]

The authors have substantially expanded this observation in a large cohort with LQTS by demonstrating that *NOS1AP* modulates QT interval and is also an independent predictor of cardiac events.[64] Therefore, genotyping *NOS1AP* is becoming an additional metric for risk stratification in LQTS (**Fig. 2**).

Modifiers in Hypertrophic Cardiomyopathy

Hints for the existence and clinical relevance of genetic modifiers in HCM have been brought to light.[65] Modifiers can be located in either known HCM genes[66] or other pathways, such as that of the rennin-angiotensin-aldosterone. Daw and colleagues[67] have mapped 4 modifier loci on 3q26.2, 10p13, 17q24, and 16q12.2 (73 cM) in a large family with HCM. The effect size of the modifier loci ranged from approximately an 8-g shift in left ventricular mass for 10p13 locus heterozygosity up to approximately 90 g for 3q26.2 locus homozygosity for the uncommon allele. Despite their early stage, these studies suggest that the clinical course of HCM may be significantly influenced by additional genetic factors.

SUMMARY

The identification of the most clinically relevant genes underlying inherited arrhythmogenic diseases and demonstration of clinical relevance of genotype-phenotype correlation require that clinical electrophysiologists are aware of the possibilities and limitations of genetic testing to squeeze out the maximum possible benefit. The authors are also facing unforeseen challenges. Genetic heterogeneity and variable expressivity of diseases hamper the risk stratification skill and reduce sensitivity and specificity of the available metrics. The findings of genetic association studies are encouraging but still require intensive research that enables to bring these results into robust clinical management algorithms. At variance with genetic association studies in the general population, this research in the field of inherited arrhythmogenic disease is made more difficult by the limited (relative to the numbers needed for this kind of studies) cohorts of patients available. This research probably requires the joint efforts from several groups of investigators, but the added values will be the availability of individualized risk profiling and clinical management.

REFERENCES

1. Bellocq C, van Ginneken AC, Bezzina CR, et al. Mutation in the KCNQ1 gene leading to the short QT-interval syndrome. Circulation 2004;109:2394–7.
2. Chen YH, Xu SJ, Bendahhou S, et al. KCNQ1 gain-of-function mutation in familial atrial fibrillation. Science 2003;299:251–4.
3. Napolitano C, Priori SG, Schwartz PJ, et al. Genetic testing in the long QT syndrome: development and validation of an efficient approach to genotyping in clinical practice. JAMA 2005;294:2975–80.
4. Tester DJ, Will ML, Haglund CM, et al. Compendium of cardiac channel mutations in 541 consecutive unrelated patients referred for long QT syndrome genetic testing. Heart Rhythm 2005;2:507–17.
5. Schwartz PJ, Priori SG, Spazzolini C, et al. Genotype-phenotype correlation in the long-QT syndrome: gene-specific triggers for life-threatening arrhythmias. Circulation 2001;103:89–95.
6. Chen L, Marquardt ML, Tester DJ, et al. Mutation of an A-kinase-anchoring protein causes long-QT syndrome. Proc Natl Acad Sci U S A 2007;104:20990–5.
7. Priori SG, Schwartz PJ, Napolitano C, et al. Risk stratification in the long-QT syndrome. N Engl J Med 2003;348:1866–74.
8. Delpon E, Cordeiro JM, Nunez L, et al. Functional effects of KCNE3 mutation and its role in the development of Brugada syndrome. Circ Arrhythm Electrophysiol 2008;1:209–18.
9. Vatta M, Ackerman MJ, Ye B, et al. Mutant caveolin-3 induces persistent late sodium current and is associated with long-QT syndrome. Circulation 2006; 114:2104–12.
10. Ueda K, Valdivia C, Medeiros-Domingo A, et al. Syntrophin mutation associated with long QT syndrome through activation of the nNOS-SCN5A macromolecular complex. Proc Natl Acad Sci U S A 2008; 105(27):9355–60.
11. London B, Michalec M, Mehdi H, et al. Mutation in glycerol-3-phosphate dehydrogenase 1 like gene (GPD1-L) decreases cardiac Na$^+$ current and causes inherited arrhythmias. Circulation 2007;116: 2260–8.
12. Watanabe H, Koopmann TT, Le Scouarnec S, et al. Sodium channel beta1 subunit mutations associated with Brugada syndrome and cardiac conduction disease in humans. J Clin Invest 2008;118: 2260–8.
13. Hu D, Martinez HI, Burashnikov E, et al. A mutation in the b3 subunit of the cardiac sodium channel associated with Brugada ECG phenotype. Circ Cardiovasc Genet 2009;2:270–8.
14. Ruan Y, Liu N, Priori SG. Sodium channel mutations and arrhythmias. Nat Rev Cardiol 2009;6:337–48.
15. Splawski I, Timothy KW, Sharpe LM, et al. Ca(V)1.2 calcium channel dysfunction causes a multisystem

disorder including arrhythmia and autism. Cell 2004; 119:19–31.

16. Bloise R, Napolitano C, Timothy KW, et al. Clinical profile and risk of sudden death in children with timothy syndrome. Circulation 2007;114(Suppl II):502.

17. Priori SG, Napolitano C. Role of genetic analyses in cardiology: part I: mendelian diseases: cardiac channelopathies. Circulation 2006;113:1130–5.

18. Antzelevitch C, Pollevick GD, Cordeiro JM, et al. Loss-of-function mutations in the cardiac calcium channel underlie a new clinical entity characterized by ST-segment elevation, short QT intervals, and sudden cardiac death. Circulation 2007;115: 442–9.

19. Yano M, Ikeda Y, Matsuzaki M. Altered intracellular Ca^{2+} handling in heart failure. J Clin Invest 2005; 115:556–64.

20. Priori SG, Napolitano C. Cardiac and skeletal muscle disorders caused by mutations in the intracellular Ca^{2+} release channels. J Clin Invest 2005; 115:2033–8.

21. Priori SG, Napolitano C, Tiso N, et al. Mutations in the cardiac ryanodine receptor gene (hRyR2) underlie catecholaminergic polymorphic ventricular tachycardia. Circulation 2001;103:196–200.

22. George CH, Jundi H, Thomas NL, et al. Ryanodine receptors and ventricular arrhythmias: emerging trends in mutations, mechanisms and therapies. J Mol Cell Cardiol 2007;42:34–50.

23. Liu N, Colombi B, Memmi M, et al. Arrhythmogenesis in catecholaminergic polymorphic ventricular tachycardia. Insights from a RyR2 R4496C knock-in mouse model. Circ Res 2006;99:292–8.

24. Lahat H, Pras E, Olender T, et al. A missense mutation in a highly conserved region of CASQ2 is associated with autosomal recessive catecholamine-induced polymorphic ventricular tachycardia in Bedouin families from Israel. Am J Hum Genet 2001;69:1378–84.

25. Rossenbacker T, Bloise R, De Giuli L, et al. Catecholaminergic polymorphic ventricular tachycardia: genetics, natural history and response to therapy. Circulation 2007;116(Suppl II):179.

26. Liu N, Rizzi N, Boveri L, et al. Ryanodine receptor and calsequestrin in arrhythmogenesis: what we have learnt from genetic diseases and transgenic mice. J Mol Cell Cardiol 2009;46:149–59.

27. Rizzi N, Liu N, Napolitano C, et al. Autosomal recessive catecholaminergic polymorphic verntricular tachycardia: pathophysiological insights from a knock-in mouse model. Circ Res 2008;103: 298–306.

28. Knollmann BC, Chopra N, Hlaing T, et al. CASQ2 deletion causes sarcoplasmic reticulum volume increase, premature Ca^{2+} release, and catecholaminergic polymorphic ventricular tachycardia. J Clin Invest 2006;116:2510–20.

29. Mohler PJ, Splawski I, Napolitano C, et al. A cardiac arrhythmia syndrome caused by loss of ankyrin-B function. Proc Natl Acad Sci U S A 2004;101: 9137–42.

30. Fowler SJ, Napolitano C, Priori SG. The genetics of cardiomyopathy: genotyping and genetic counseling. Curr Treat Options Cardiovasc Med 2009; 11:433–46.

31. Sen-Chowdhry S, Syrris P, McKenna WJ. Role of genetic analysis in the management of patients with arrhythmogenic right ventricular dysplasia/ cardiomyopathy. J Am Coll Cardiol 2007;50: 1813–21.

32. Beffagna G, Occhi G, Nava A, et al. Regulatory mutations in transforming growth factor-beta3 gene cause arrhythmogenic right ventricular cardiomyopathy type 1. Cardiovasc Res 2005;65:366–73.

33. Niimura H, Bachinski LL, Sangwatanaroj S, et al. Mutations in the gene for cardiac myosin-binding protein C and late-onset familial hypertrophic cardiomyopathy. N Engl J Med 1998;338:1248–57.

34. Richard P, Charron P, Carrier L, et al. Hypertrophic cardiomyopathy: distribution of disease genes, spectrum of mutations, and implications for a molecular diagnosis strategy. Circulation 2003;107:2227–32.

35. Maron BJ, Spirito P, Shen WK, et al. Implantable cardioverter-defibrillators and prevention of sudden cardiac death in hypertrophic cardiomyopathy. JAMA 2007;298:405–12.

36. Juang JM, Chern YR, Tsai CT, et al. The association of human connexin 40 genetic polymorphisms with atrial fibrillation. Int J Cardiol 2007;116(1):107–12.

37. Gudbjartsson DF, Arnar DO, Helgadottir A, et al. Variants conferring risk of atrial fibrillation on chromosome 4q25. Nature 2007;448:353–7.

38. Wadelius M, Chen LY, Lindh JD, et al. The largest prospective warfarin-treated cohort supports genetic forecasting. Blood 2009;113:784–92.

39. Priori SG, Napolitano C, Schwartz PJ, et al. Association of long QT syndrome loci and cardiac events among patients treated with beta-blockers. JAMA 2004;292:1341–4.

40. Mok NS, Priori SG, Napolitano C, et al. A newly characterized SCN5A mutation underlying Brugada syndrome unmasked by hyperthermia. J Cardiovasc Electrophysiol 2003;14:407–11.

41. Napolitano C, Schwartz PJ, Brown AM, et al. Evidence for a cardiac ion channel mutation underlying drug-induced QT prolongation and life-threatening arrhythmias. J Cardiovasc Electrophysiol 2000;11:691–6.

42. Zipes DP, Camm AJ, Borggrefe M, et al. ACC/AHA/ ESC 2006 guidelines for management of patients with ventricular arrhythmias and the prevention of sudden cardiac death: a report of the American College of Cardiology/American Heart Association

Task Force and the European Society of Cardiology Committee for Practice Guidelines (writing committee to develop guidelines for management of patients with ventricular arrhythmias and the prevention of sudden cardiac death): developed in collaboration with the European Heart Rhythm Association and the Heart Rhythm Society. Circulation 2006;114:e385–484.

43. Kapa S, Tester DJ, Salisbury BA, et al. Genetic testing for long-QT syndrome: distinguishing pathogenic mutations from benign variants. Circulation 2009;120:1752–60.

44. Moss AJ, Shimizu W, Wilde AA, et al. Clinical aspects of type-1 long-QT syndrome by location, coding type, and biophysical function of mutations involving the KCNQ1 gene. Circulation 2007;115:2481–9.

45. Benhorin J, Taub R, Goldmit M, et al. Effects of flecainide in patients with new SCN5A mutation: mutation-specific therapy for long-QT syndrome? Circulation 2000;101:1698–706.

46. Ruan Y, Liu N, Bloise R, et al. Gating properties of SCN5A mutations and the response to mexiletine in long-QT syndrome type 3 patients. Circulation 2007;116:1137–44.

47. Ruan Y, Denegri M, Liu N, et al. Trafficking defects and gating abnormalities of a novel SCN5A mutation question gene-specific therapy in long QT syndrome type 3. Circ Res 2010;106:1374–83.

48. Ingles J, Doolan A, Chiu C, et al. Compound and double mutations in patients with hypertrophic cardiomyopathy: implications for genetic testing and counseling. J Med Genet 2005;42:e59.

49. Keren A, Syrris P, McKenna WJ. Hypertrophic cardiomyopathy: the genetic determinants of clinical disease expression. Nat Clin Pract Cardiovasc Med 2008;5:747.

50. Bauce B, Nava A, Beffagna G, et al. Multiple mutations in desmosomal proteins encoding genes in arrhythmogenic right ventricular cardiomyopathy/dysplasia. Heart Rhythm 2010;7:22–9.

51. Westenskow P, Splawski I, Timothy KW, et al. Compound mutations: a common cause of severe long-QT syndrome. Circulation 2004;109:1834–41.

52. Kobori A, Sarai N, Shimizu W, et al. Additional gene variants reduce effectiveness of beta-blockers in the LQT1 form of long QT syndrome. J Cardiovasc Electrophysiol 2004;15:190–9.

53. Arking DE, Pfeufer A, Post W, et al. A common genetic variant in the NOS1 regulator NOS1AP modulates cardiac repolarization. Nat Genet 2006;38:644–51.

54. Pfeufer A, Sanna S, Arking DE, et al. Common variants at ten loci modulate the QT interval duration in the QTSCD Study. Nat Genet 2009;41:407–14.

55. Smith JG, Lowe JK, Kovvali S, et al. Genome-wide association study of electrocardiographic conduction measures in an isolated founder population: Kosrae. Heart Rhythm 2009;6:634–41.

56. Marroni F, Pfeufer A, Aulchenko YS, et al. A genome-wide association scan of RR and QT interval duration in 3 European genetically isolated populations: the EUROSPAN Project. Circ Cardiovasc Genet 2009;2:322–8.

57. Wilton SB, Anderson TJ, Parboosingh J, et al. Polymorphisms in multiple genes are associated with resting heart rate in a stepwise allele-dependent manner. Heart Rhythm 2008;5:694–700.

58. Crotti L, Lundquist AL, Insolia R, et al. KCNH2-K897T is a genetic modifier of latent congenital long-QT syndrome. Circulation 2005;112:1251–8.

59. Tan BH, Valdivia CR, Rok BA, et al. Common human SCN5A polymorphisms have altered electrophysiology when expressed in Q1077 splice variants. Heart Rhythm 2005;2:741–7.

60. Gui J, Wang T, Trump D, et al. Mutation-specific effects of polymorphism H558R in SCN5A-related sick sinus syndrome. J Cardiovasc Electrophysiol 2010;21(5):564–73.

61. Bezzina CR, Verkerk AO, Busjahn A, et al. A common polymorphism in KCNH2 (HERG) hastens cardiac repolarization. Cardiovasc Res 2003;59:27–36.

62. Chang KC, Barth AS, Sasano T, et al. CAPON modulates cardiac repolarization via neuronal nitric oxide synthase signaling in the heart. Proc Natl Acad Sci U S A 2008;105:4477–82.

63. Crotti L, Monti MC, Insolia R, et al. NOS1AP is a genetic modifier of the long-QT syndrome. Circulation 2009;120:1657–63.

64. Tomas M, Napolitano C, De Giuli L, et al. Polymorphisms in the NOS1AP gene modulate QT interval duration and risk of arrhythmias in the long QT syndrome. J Am Coll Cardiol 2010;55(24):2745–52.

65. Marian AJ. Genetic determinants of cardiac hypertrophy. Curr Opin Cardiol 2008;23:199–205.

66. Wang P, Zou Y, Fu C, et al. MYBPC3 polymorphism is a modifier for expression of cardiac hypertrophy in patients with hypertrophic cardiomyopathy. Biochem Biophys Res Commun 2005;329:796–9.

67. Daw EW, Chen SN, Czernuszewicz G, et al. Genome-wide mapping of modifier chromosomal loci for human hypertrophic cardiomyopathy. Hum Mol Genet 2007;16:2463–71.

Index

Card Electrophysiol Clin 2 (2010) 635–638
doi:10.1016/S1877-9182(10)00156-5
1877-9182/10/$ – see front matter

cardiacEP.theclinics.com

Printed and bound by CPI Group (UK) Ltd, Croydon, CR0 4YY

03/10/2024

01040357-0016